THE **COMPLETE IDIOT'S GUIDE** TO

Chakras

by Betsy Rippentrop, Ph.D., and Eve Adamson

ALPHA

A member of Penguin Group (USA) Inc.

This book is for our children—Pieter, Jack, Angus, and Emmett—and all other children, that they may learn to be strong, confident, tender, and loving, with healthy bodies, free emotions, open minds, and loving spirits. That is our wish for you, too, as you continue in your quest to be your best self. The human race is evolving to the next level and you are helping to effect that change through your own inner work. We honor the light within you. Namaste.

ALPHA BOOKS

Published by the Penguin Group

Penguin Group (USA) Inc., 375 Hudson Street, New York, New York 10014, USA

Penguin Group (Canada), 90 Eglinton Avenue East, Suite 700, Toronto, Ontario M4P 2Y3, Canada (a division of Pearson Penguin Canada Inc.)

Penguin Books Ltd., 80 Strand, London WC2R 0RL, England

Penguin Ireland, 25 St. Stephen's Green, Dublin 2, Ireland (a division of Penguin Books Ltd.)

Penguin Group (Australia), 250 Camberwell Road, Camberwell, Victoria 3124, Australia (a division of Pearson Australia Group Pty. Ltd.)

Penguin Books India Pvt. Ltd., 11 Community Centre, Panchsheel Park, New Delhi—110 017, India

Penguin Group (NZ), 67 Apollo Drive, Rosedale, North Shore, Auckland 1311, New Zealand (a division of Pearson New Zealand Ltd.)

Penguin Books (South Africa) (Pty.) Ltd., 24 Sturdee Avenue, Rosebank, Johannesburg 2196, South Africa

Penguin Books Ltd., Registered Offices: 80 Strand, London WC2R 0RL, England

Publisher: *Marie Butler-Knight*
Editorial Director: *Mike Sanders*
Senior Managing Editor: *Billy Fields*
Executive Editor: *Randy Ladenheim-Gil*
Book Producer: *Lee Ann Chearney/Amaranth IlluminAre*
Development Editor: *Ginny Bess Munroe*
Senior Production Editor: *Megan Douglass*
Copy Editor: *Emily Garner*

Cartoonist: *Steve Barr*
Illustrations: *Wendy Frost*
Cover Designer: *Bill Thomas*
Book Designer: *Trina Wurst*
Indexer: *Brad Herriman*
Layout: *Ayanna Lacey*
Proofreader: *John Etchison*

Contents at a Glance

Appendixes

Contents

Appendixes

Introduction

You know who you are. You've looked in the mirror thousands of times. You've got a name, physical qualities, things you do. People you know recognize you when they see you. But what's going on *inside?* Is there more to you than you can see in that mirror, more than your friends and family know, more than even you have dreamed?

You *are* more than just a body. You are a confluence of energies, like a network of rivers and streams burgeoning with life. You are part of something bigger, and yet, you are also ultimately a unique, individual spirit. Don't worry if you don't see it all just yet. You've got a secret code, a key inside you that can guide you toward greater self-realization. You've got chakras. In ancient Sanskrit, the word *chakra* means "wheel," and these seven spinning energy vortexes inside your body, located along your spine from the bottom of your pelvis to the crown of your head, reveal more about you than any reflection or description ever could. Your chakras constantly open and close, widen and narrow, turn and spin, taking in and releasing life force energy according to *your* life, *your* experiences, and who you are at any given moment. They are wheels of light and they are all about you. Get to know them, and you get to know yourself.

We've written this book to help you make the most of the chakras you hold inside you. We are Dr. Betsy Rippentrop and Eve Adamson. What do we know about chakras? Betsy is a licensed psychologist, hypnotherapist, and Reiki practitioner, as well as an Anusara yoga teacher-in-training. Betsy uses the chakras in her psychology practice to help her clients better understand themselves and heal. She measures clients' chakras early in treatment to serve as a baseline, and routinely monitors clients' chakras throughout treatment to help them understand their patterns and progress. She'll show you how to measure your chakras, too. Betsy also utilizes her chakra knowledge to help her yoga students understand the subtle energies in their bodies, and how yoga can help neutralize imbalances they may have.

Your other co-author Eve Adamson is a writer and devoted yoga practitioner who checks in almost daily with her own chakras, to get a better sense of why she is feeling, for example, imbalanced, assertive, moody, or particularly insightful on any particular day. Together, we will guide you through your own chakras, introducing you and helping you get to know them better. We'll show you how to use them, how to decode the messages they write in your physical body, and how to keep in touch with yourself through these spinning centers of your own life force. Hip pain? Neck pain? Fallen arches or sore throat? Sudden sadness or unexplained joy? The answers lie within those spinning wheels.

This is a journey of self-knowledge—one that can catapult you to the next level of your personal evolution.

Throughout this book, we also discuss how blocks and overloads in our chakras may lead to certain physical and/or mental health problems. We acknowledge that many factors come into play regarding a person's likelihood of developing illness or disease (i.e., genetics, lifestyle, diet, weight). Yet we believe that when chakras are out of balance for extended periods of time, this energy disparity increases the likelihood of developing disease. If you break apart the word disease, it actually becomes dis-ease, or a lack of ease, a lack of balance.

Nobody wants to become ill, but disease and illness are opportunities, even if they don't feel that way. This is your body's way of alerting you, of protecting you, of telling you that something is off-kilter and needs to be addressed. If you have a disease or health condition, there is no blame here. You have been doing the best you can in your life with the information you had. You are now receiving new information from your body, in the form of symptoms. Use this new information to improve your life, to seek balance, to take better care of yourself, to acknowledge and understand your fears, and to release any anger or resentment you've been carrying. Our bodies are extremely wise, and will give us the signs we need. A better life is waiting if we are willing and brave enough to explore the meaning behind the symptoms, and that exploration can begin with the chakras.

Are you ready to be self-realized, empowered, and more at home than ever before in your own body, mind, and spirit? Are you ready to integrate all the parts of yourself into one amazing whole? Then you are ready to start working with your chakras. So grab the wheel, and get ready to start driving your own life. You've got an exciting journey ahead, and we'll be right there with you.

About This Book

The Complete Idiot's Guide to Chakras is divided into five parts that cover everything you need to know to explore and balance your own chakras.

In **Part 1, "All About the Chakras,"** we introduce you to the whole chakra concept, from a brief explanation of each chakra, where it is, and what it means, to a fun history lesson about chakras and an explanation about how they actually work in the body, in conjunction with the entire network of life force energy.

In **Part 2, "Dynamics of Chakra Force,"** we explore all the many symbolic examples of chakras, from the tiniest atom to the largest galaxy. In this part, you'll learn about the notorious *Kundalini* energy so critical to understanding chakra awakening, and you'll also learn how to work with your actual chakras, including how to measure them.

Part 3, **"Know Your Chakras: Bottoms Up!,"** is the heart of the book. We spend a chapter on each of the seven chakras, telling you everything you need to know about what each one means, what happens when it gets blocked or overloaded with energy, and how to heal and balance it.

In **Part 4, "High Octane Bliss ... No Caffeine Necessary!,"** we get serious about actually integrating chakra work into real life, with chapters on using chakras to feel better every day, using your own voice to increase chakra vibration, how chakras can enhance your love life, and how to use meditation techniques for greater chakra awareness.

Part 5, **"Relax, Release, Restore, Renew,"** covers more advanced techniques for working with the chakras, from partner exercises for releasing chakra blocks to guided visualizations and an exploration of the astral and causal bodies.

Extras

Throughout each chapter in this book, you'll find four types of extra information, nicely bundled into little boxes for your reading pleasure. These add to your practical knowledge, filling you in on all those weird words we tend to use, telling you stories about us or about Betsy's clients, and helping you out with things you can do, or things you shouldn't do, for greater chakra power.

!!! Wake-Up Call

These are the things to watch out for, to help you avoid and solve any problems you might have as you navigate your chakras.

def•i•ni•tion

What the heck are we talking about? These boxes decipher those Sanskrit words, medical terms, and other jargon.

Spinning Your Wheels

We've got a million stories, and we tell you some of them here, about Betsy's clients (all names and identifying details have been changed) and about ourselves and our own experiences, when we think they might help you out.

Energy Unplugged

These boxes are full of advice or practical tips about things you can actually do to help open, balance, or heal your chakras. These are your to-do boxes.

Acknowledgments

Betsy: Thanks to Eve Adamson for being my experienced, wise, and grounded guide who journeyed with me on this amazing chakra trip! Thanks to Dr. Candida Maurer and Dr. Michael Santangelo, who first opened my eyes to the world of energy, chakras, Reiki, and healing—your wisdom and guidance have been priceless. Thanks to Marsha Nieland, my Anusara teacher and mentor, for changing my life by your strong practice, exceptional teaching, open heart, playfulness, generosity, and dedication to the kula. Thanks to all the exceptional teachers who work with me at Heartland Yoga—this studio would not be thriving without your talents and enthusiasm. Thanks to my boys: Pieter, for constant comic relief, grounding, and reminding me of what is truly important in life; and Jack, my steady, stable, and blissful baby boy who epitomizes open-heartedness. Finally, this book is dedicated to my dear husband, Jon, who always lends his support and believes in me, no matter what adventure I'm navigating.

Eve: Thank you to my fantastic, loving, open-hearted co-author, Dr. Betsy Rippentrop, whose beautiful spirit and trusty expertise trickles down through every page of this book. Thanks to my BFF and fellow yogi Rachel Klapper, who was a behind-the-scenes source of help, information, and moral support during the writing of this book. Thanks to Lee Ann, for bringing me this wonderful project, which I enjoyed so much. Thanks to my youngest son, Emmett, who patiently let me measure his chakras and test visualizations and meditations on him. He's only 10 but he's a wise spirit filled with love and compassion. He has a magnificent Heart chakra. And as always, thanks to Ben, for listening, for keeping the kids out of the office when I was under deadline, for letting the dogs out so I wouldn't have to break my train of thought, and for making sure there was food on the table (even if it was meat) when I was unable to do even one more thing. I couldn't do this job without you, babe!

Trademarks

Part 1

All About the Chakras

You've heard about them. You've seen pictures. Maybe you've even felt them. But just what are your chakras, where are they, and what do they mean for you and your life? This part has all the answers. You'll find an at-a-glance chart along with introductory information about each chakra and how it influences your body, mind, and spirit. Learn about chakra history (painless, we promise!), then discover a whole new way of looking at your own anatomy, moving beyond bones, muscles, and internal organs to exam *prana*, *nadis*, and the way energy moves in, out, and through your body and its energy centers.

Where Are Your Chakras?

In This Chapter

- ◆ What chakras are and what they mean to you
- ◆ How you already know your own chakras
- ◆ Chakras one through seven: an overview
- ◆ What a chakra isn't, so you can quit worrying
- ◆ Making your chakras work for you

Do you ever wonder why on some days you feel safe, secure, and calm, as if all is right with the world, whereas on other days you feel jittery and anxious, as if someone is about to pull the rug out from under you?

Do you ever notice how on some days you feel so emotional that you can hardly keep yourself from giggling aloud or bursting into tears, whereas on other days you frankly don't care … about anything?

Have you ever thought of someone just before they happen to call you on the phone or send you an e-mail, or have you ever started singing a popular song just before it comes on the radio?

And whether or not you consider yourself a spiritual or religious person, do you ever wonder why you have those occasional uplifting moments of realization, those *a-ha* moments that make you feel like you just might be directly connected to some higher power?

All those feelings are natural, normal, and part of being human, but they also come from somewhere. They come straight out of your body. To be more precise, they flow from your very own energy-infused, rainbow-hued, spinning *chakras*.

How You've Already Touched Your Chakras

If you picked up this book, you've probably heard about and want to learn more about chakras, even if you aren't exactly sure what they are. You may already assume you *have* chakras, and you might even know they are stacked up in line with your backbone, from the base of your spine to the crown of your head.

You might have heard that you have five, or seven, or eight, or even hundreds of chakras. Or maybe you have no idea how many might be spinning around inside you. Have you heard that chakras spin? The word chakra means "wheel" in Sanskrit, and that's exactly what these energy vortexes are: spinning wheels of energy—*your* energy.

def•i•ni•tion

According to ancient Indian wisdom, **chakras** (pronounced cha-kra, with a hard "ch" like in "chair") are spinning energy centers in the body that lie along the body's many energy pathways. While chakras correspond to certain glands, nerve centers, and organs in the body, they are part of the subtle energy body, not the physical body, so they cannot be detected by standard medical equipment such as x-rays or MRIs. Chakras also correspond to various aspects of the body's physical, psychological, emotional, and spiritual state

Even if you don't know much about chakras, we can guarantee that you have already felt them. A nervous stomach when you have to do something brave is your third chakra talking. The lump in your throat when you have something important to say but have trouble getting it out is your fifth chakra in action. Those lower-down butterflies you get when you see, touch, or even think about your romantic partner live in your second chakra. That constipation you get when you are traveling far from home is your first chakra getting protective. That stabbing pain in your heart when someone has broken it? That's your injured and throbbing fourth chakra.

You may have also been aware of your chakras while engaging in some of the holistic practices that tap into them, such as yoga, energy healing (like Reiki), or massage. A doctor can't pinpoint a chakra, but that doesn't mean you don't feel your heart opening up when you do a deep back-bend, or feel calm and grounded after a massage, or have a sudden insight after an energy healer has set your *prana* or your *chi* flowing more freely again.

def•i•ni•tion

Many of the words having to do with the chakras come from **Sanskrit,** an ancient literary language from India. **Prana** is the Sanskrit term for life force energy, which flows into and out of the body with the breath and through the chakras via channels in the body called *nadis.* **Chi** is the Chinese term for the same life force energy, and is the term acupuncturists, Shiatsu massage therapists, and other energy healers often use. *Prana* and *chi* are essentially the same thing, going by different names because they come from different languages. Because the word chakra is a Sanskrit word, in this book, we generally use the term *prana* instead of *chi* when talking about this life force energy.

But so what if you have chakras, and so what if you feel them? What does it mean for you? It can mean plenty if you learn to read your own chakras, because they can tell you a lot, not only about who you are, but about how you can increase your health, balance your emotions, clear your mind, improve your relationships, feel more powerful, and even have a more fulfilling spiritual life. Understanding your chakras can greatly increase the speed of your personal evolution as they increase your self-awareness and ability to grow and change in positive ways. You'll "get" yourself better than ever before. So what are you waiting for?

The Wheels Are Turning

Chakras are an amazing tool in your own body, to help you get to know and understand yourself better. They are like a barometer for your internal weather—a measure of who you are at any given moment.

Chakras provide a template for your entire life, with each chakra governing major aspects of who you are (your first chakra), how you feel (your second chakra), what you do (your third chakra), how you love (your fourth chakra), what you say (your fifth chakra), what you know (your sixth chakra), and how you perceive your connection with the universe or a higher power (your seventh chakra).

Throughout this book, we'll explore each chakra and how you can learn about and use yours, but just to get you started thinking about your own chakras, check out the following table to see what each chakra does, in brief.

	Common name	Sanskrit name	Location	Associated color	Element	Associated physiology	Influences/Energy
First Chakra	Root chakra	*Muladhara* (meaning "root")	Base of the spine	Red	Earth	Feet, legs, hips, bones, joints, sacrum, coccygeal nerve plexus, Lower intestine, waste removal system	Security, safety, survival, basic needs (food and shelter), grounding, family and tribe, and health
Second chakra	Sacral chakra	*Svadhisthana* (meaning "dwelling place of the self" or "sweetness")	Just below the navel	Orange	Water	Reproductive organs, sacral nerve plexus, lower back, pelvis, abdomen, bladder	Emotions, movement, feelings, pleasure, sexuality, fertility, and creativity
Third chakra	Solar Plexus chakra	*Manipura* (meaning "dwelling place for the jewel" or "city of the jewel"	At the solar plexus, at the base of the rib cage	Yellow	Fire	Stomach, digestive organs, adrenal glands, liver, kidney, spleen, pancreas, middle back, solar nerve plexus	Power, energy, self-esteem, will, ego/sense of self, taking action, and making things happen

Common name	Sanskrit name	Location	Associated color	Element	Associated physiology	Influences/Energy
Fourth chakra	Heart chakra	*Anahata* (meaning "intact" or "unstruck"—the place that sings without being played)	Behind the heart	Green	Air	Thymus gland, cardiac nerve plexus, heart, lungs, shoulders, arms, breasts	Love, compassion, empathy, kindness, balance, quest for peace, and love of self
Fifth chakra	Throat chakra	*Vissudha* (meaning "purity")	Behind the throat, at the base of the neck	Bright blue	Sound	Throat, trachea, neck, thyroid gland, pharyngeal nerve plexus, mouth	Communication, speaking the truth, listening, hearing the truth, metaphorical thinking, and manifesting creativity
Sixth chakra	Third Eye chakra	*Ajna* (meaning "understanding" or "commanding")	On the forehead, about an inch above the brow line	Deep indigo	Light	Pituitary and pineal glands, carotid nerve plexus	Intuition, imagination, perception, dreams, symbolic thinking, inner wisdom, and psychic vision
Seventh chakra	Crown chakra	*Sahasrara* (meaning "thousand")	At the crown of the head	Purple	Thought	Brain, nervous system, pituitary and pineal glands, cerebral cortex	Spirituality, intelligence, connection to a higher power, broad-mindedness, divinity, union, and seeing the "big picture"

Your Body, Your Chakras

If you decided you wanted to look back into the history of Indian philosophy and theology for information on the chakras, you would find it—but some information would contradict other information you might find. Some traditions say the chakras are five regions of the body. Some systems pinpoint hundreds of chakras. Although many different sub-traditions have evaluated and interpreted the chakras in different ways, for the purposes of this book, we use the model most commonly accepted today: the seven-chakra system. This system says we have seven energy centers that run along the midline of the body from the base of the spine to the crown of the head. We acknowledge that there are other, smaller chakras in other parts of the body, most notably in the hands and feet, and sometimes we make note of those, especially in the way the foot chakras can help ground you via your first chakra, and the way the hand chakras can help heal you via the fourth chakra. But we get into all that later.

For now, let's take a brief look at the seven primary chakras, where they are, and what they mean for you. We cover each chakra in more detail in Part 3 of this book, but the following sections get you started. Consider it a formal introduction to your own chakra system.

The First Chakra

First chakra.

Call it the Root chakra, the Earth chakra, the Foundation chakra, or use the official Sanskrit term: *Muladhara chakra*. The first chakra is located at the base of your spine, in front of your tailbone. Its symbolic color is red and its symbolic element is Earth. This chakra is also the center for your feelings of safety, survival, and security, and the very root and foundation of your physical body. It all starts here.

When your first chakra is healthy and open, you feel a sense of connection to the earth, you feel comfortable in your own body, and you feel safe. You feel physically healthy, financially secure, and you have a strong sense of self. You know who you are and where you belong.

If your first chakra is too tightly closed, you feel flighty and untethered. You are too much in your head, or too swayed by your emotions. You aren't sure what home is, or you feel lost. You sometimes feel like you might just float away into the sky because you don't really feel like you belong anywhere. You may have trouble managing your money or practicing good health habits. You might even get so distracted by your thoughts or strong feelings or even by spiritual practices like meditation or prayer that you forget to do basic survival things like pay your bills, brush your teeth, or eat your dinner. You might tend to trip a lot, have trouble balancing in yoga poses, or twist your ankles, or you may have foot or hip pain.

On the other hand, if your first chakra is too wide open, you may be sluggish, have trouble moving very much, feel heavy and earthbound, or have a hard time getting things done. You might be a homebody to your own detriment, refusing to leave home or take any risks that involve change and movement. You might also feel ruled by your basic instincts, rather than being in charge of them—your hunger, thirst, desire for sleep, or need to exercise may be so strong that they keep you from getting other things done or interacting with other people. People who overeat, sleep too much, or are addicted to exercise sometimes have first-chakra issues, although those problems can also be related to other chakras. (Most issues people have involve more than one chakra, but we get into that more later.)

Our goal is to get your first chakra up and running, strong, healthy, and balanced with the other chakras. This chakra is an important one because all the others stand on top of it. While some people think spiritual pursuits are somehow "higher" or "better" than physical pursuits, we argue that without a strong foundation in the first chakra, it is hard to develop the higher chakras. Right now, you live in the world, in a body, and your job is to do that as well as you can. Your first chakra gives you the power and the resources to do that.

The Second Chakra

Second chakra.

The second chakra is sometimes called the Sacral chakra, Sex chakra, or Emotion chakra. The Sanskrit term for this chakra is *Svadhisthana*. Its symbolic color is orange, its symbolic element is water, and it is the center of emotions, feelings, creativity, movement, and sexuality. While feelings of love and compassion originate in the fourth or Heart chakra, the second chakra is the source of passion, desire, sexual attraction, and sexual relationships. Your creativity comes from here, and for women, you create *life* here, as the second chakra is also the seat of your fertility.

When you have a strong, healthy, open second chakra, you are comfortable with your emotions and can feel them strongly without letting them take over (a strong first chakra will help, too). Your creativity flows and you have the ability to get things done, make things happen, and accept changes in life with grace and ease. A strong second chakra also fuels a healthy sex life and helps you feel sexy, desirable, and satisfied. You aren't afraid to feel things. When you get butterflies in your stomach, you are feeling your second chakra. This is your pleasure center.

If, on the other hand, your second chakra is closed, your emotions may feel cut off or blocked. You may appear cold or unfeeling to others, even though on the inside your emotions are a mix of depression and frustration. Physically, people with closed second chakras might experience infertility, sexual problems, chronic pelvic pain, gynecological problems, and prostate cancer. If you have trouble finishing things, fear progress, feel disconnected from your creativity, or have trouble enjoying sex, you may have a second chakra block. Your second chakra might also be closed if you don't or can't feel intimately bonded with your romantic partner. (Although the problem may be related to your partner's second chakra issues, in most cases, both second chakras are involved when a couple has intimacy issues or doesn't feel emotionally bonded.) To protect a sensitive and closed second chakra, some people also gain excess weight in their abdomen.

If your second chakra is too open, you are ruled by your emotions and they sometimes keep you from getting anything done. You feel *too* strongly, so that it becomes incapacitating. Sexual addiction can also be related to a too-open second chakra (although ironically, it can be related to a too-closed second chakra, too, if you are addicted to sex without emotional involvement). An overly large second chakra can also result in addictions and hedonism without discipline or structure.

Ideally, you can balance your second chakra with your first chakra. If you have a strong, grounded foundation, then you will feel more able to experience your emotions safely and freely.

The Third Chakra

Third chakra.

The third chakra, sometimes called the Solar Plexus chakra, Power chakra, or in Sanskrit, *Manipura,* is the seat of your personal power. Its color is sunny yellow, and its element is fire. Confident people radiate like the sun from the third chakra, projecting their energy in front of them from this spot over the solar plexus. This chakra is also linked with your digestion and the transformation of food to energy. What you take in here, you radiate out to the world.

If your third chakra is too closed, you will tend to feel powerless, as if you are at the mercy of fate (or other people) and have no control over what happens to you. Weak third chakras often result in victim mentality, lack of willpower, and an inability to be effective. Digestive problems also originate here, such as irritable bowel syndrome, indigestion, and constipation. A poor appetite and disinterest in food may also be related to the third chakra, as well as weight gain, as if your body is trying to pad and protect your third chakra with body fat (this can also happen when your body tries to protect your sensitive second chakra).

A too-open third chakra can be related to over-aggressiveness, bossiness, self-centeredness (narcissism), and being overly strict, both with yourself and with others. Very dominant, loud people with huge energy who take over a room often have third chakras that are too open. They may get things done, but at the expense of others, especially if they have a closed fourth chakra at the same time. Sometimes it can feel like these people are shooting others down with the intense power of their third chakras.

When you balance your third chakra with the others, you can radiate your personal power and have a strong, confident sense of who you are without stepping on others or ignoring your own feelings and intuitions. A balanced third chakra is effectively powerful and courageous, with a healthy dose of humility.

The Fourth Chakra

The fourth chakra is usually known as the Heart chakra. In Sanskrit, it is called *Anahata.* This chakra's color is green and its element is air. The Heart chakra is just what it sounds like it is: the place from which you love. This is also the middle chakra—the three chakras below it are generally considered to be the earthly chakras, and the three chakras above it are generally considered to be the spiritual chakras. The heart links both sides together and anchors them into *you.* Your heart keeps your physical, earthly qualities in balance with your spiritual, more ethereal qualities, so that you can have both a spiritual life and an earthly body. It all hangs together because of love, which—according to chakra philosophy—is the very fuel for existence.

Fourth chakra.

When your fourth chakra is closed, you have a hard time loving. You may feel like you've never really been in love, or your love relationships feel shallow. You might have trouble sympathizing with others, or feeling empathy. You might also have dif-ficulty feeling love toward yourself. If your third chakra (just below the fourth) is simultaneously too open, you may be more concerned with power and success and yourself than with others. If your fifth chakra (just above the fourth) is simultaneously too open, you may be more interested in intellectual talking than in actual compassion for what's going on right in front of you. Because the fourth chakra is *so essential* for linking body, mind, and spirit into an integrated whole, many yoga poses are intensely focused on opening this chakra, often through backbends. Closed fourth chakras can also be related to actual heart disease, specifically heart attacks, angina, and other con-ditions related to clogged and blocked arteries to the heart.

When the fourth chakra is too open, you may have a martyr complex: you feel so compelled to help others and sacrifice your own needs for the needs of humanity that you neglect yourself completely. You might lose your grounding or your sense of personal power because all you care about is giving yourself away. You might also feel such strong empathy for the feelings of others that you mistake those feelings for your own and lose your sense of identity.

When you learn to balance your fourth chakra with the other chakras, you can love fully, openly, and sincerely. You also feel comfortable accepting the sense of deep inner peace that true compassion and the ability to love can bring to your body, mind, and spirit. Your fourth chakra serves as an anchor for all the other chakras, yoking them together like a strong central link in a long chain.

The Fifth Chakra

Fifth chakra.

The fifth chakra, or Throat chakra, is called *Vishuddha* in Sanskrit. Its color is a bright sapphire blue, and its element is sound. The fifth chakra produces your voice and is the center for creative expression. When you talk, write, even draw or paint, that impulse comes from here—it is the place that compels you to communicate your ideas about the world. The fifth chakra is also the truth center. From here, you can speak the truth, and you can also learn to hear the truth from others, rather than deluding yourself about what is happening.

A closed fifth chakra can result in a hard time communicating. You might stumble over words, stutter, or tend to be silent, even when it would be appropriate to speak. You may know exactly what you want to say,

Energy Unplugged

The fifth chakra is about speaking, but also about writing and drawing. When you are having trouble getting to the core issue of a problem or discovering the truth of a situation, try writing your random thoughts or even drawing a picture. The answer might pop out and surprise you, courtesy of your fifth chakra.

but just can't get the words out. Often, you fear telling people what you really believe and become good at literally "swallowing" your words. You might also have a compulsion to lie, or to lie to yourself that what you are saying is true. A closed fifth chakra also makes it difficult to hear the truth, especially the truth beyond the actual words someone else might be saying. You may experience creative blocks, like writer's block, or feel as if you can't find inspiration. Physically, you might experience sore throats, laryngitis, neck pain, and ear infections. Most of us have felt a temporarily closed fifth chakra in the form of a lump in the throat, when we are trying not to say something or trying to repress a strong emotion that wants to come out in words or sobbing.

People with fifth chakras that are too open often tend to talk too much, yammering on long after it is time to listen. Being in a relationship with someone like this can be exhausting because they don't stop talking and they rarely listen. Although such people may be prolific creators, they may be so intellectually stimulated that they lose sight of other people's feelings or needs. If you attack others with words, argue incessantly, dominate conversations, always have to prove your point to be right, or are so focused on what to say next instead of actually listening, your fifth chakra is probably too open.

A balanced fifth chakra taps into the heart below and the intuition above to speak and hear the truth in just the right measure, so you can be creatively charged but also socially sensitive.

The Sixth Chakra

Sixth chakra.

The sixth chakra is the Third Eye chakra, or *Ajna* in Sanskrit. Its color is a deep indigo or, according to some systems, a deep royal purple, and its element is light. The sixth chakra is the center of your intuition—that feeling you get when you just *know* something is true, even though you have no physical evidence. Your sixth chakra picks up on cues your conscious mind doesn't necessarily detect. It governs your inner knowledge of both yourself and the world. Some people attribute clairvoyance, or psychic "seeing," to this chakra, while others believe clairvoyance is just a more refined and sensitive ability to see. This is the place to cultivate that skill.

If you have a closed sixth chakra, you are more likely to be oblivious to your own inner wisdom. You ignore—or don't even hear—those prodding urges that tell you to cross to the other side of the street or accept an offer or ask a friend if something is wrong. You may live too much in your body and be too entrenched in your physical life to spend much time on inner contemplation and the cultivation of your sixth sense, especially if you have an overly open first chakra. Or, if you have an overly open second or fourth chakra, your own emotions or the emotions and needs of others might cloud your inner judgment and ability to see the big picture. People with closed sixth chakras also might experience sinus headaches, tension headaches, sinus infections, near-sightedness, and other vision problems.

Having a too-open sixth chakra can make you feel ungrounded in reality. People with sixth chakras that are too open tend to be too much in their head, overly intellectual, and likely to overthink everything. If your sixth chakra is too open, you may also confuse your dreams with your waking reality or even see visions and be unsure whether they are real. Such people often are so caught up in spiritual pursuits or psychic "seeing" that they forget they are in human bodies, living a human life.

If you think you have psychic abilities, see ghosts, and/or spend a lot of time meditating, you need to be particularly careful to nurture and strengthen your lower chakras. A balanced sixth chakra enables you to tap into inner knowing and wisdom, both in the world and within yourself, while also remaining grounded in the world and in your body. This balance also enables you to temper your strong intellect with emotion and heart.

The Seventh Chakra

The seventh chakra, sometimes called the Crown chakra or the Thousand-Petaled Lotus chakra, is called *Sahasrara* in Sanskrit. Its color is purple, or according to some systems, pure white. Its element is thought. The Crown chakra is the seat of pure consciousness, wisdom, and enlightenment. Here lies your universal self, the self that is greater than the individual you. A healthy seventh chakra indicates a healthy spiritual life and an awareness that you are connected with all things. There is some of you in everyone and everything else, and some of everyone and everything else in you. Spirit, divinity, God, Goddess, or whatever you consider to be the source of all creation and the key to enlightenment, speaks to you through this chakra, and lives inside you through this chakra.

Seventh chakra.

People with closed seventh chakras have no interest in spiritual pursuits, may be atheists, and make materialism and their own needs priorities. People with closed seventh chakras probably would never seek out holistic healers, nor would they be likely to pick up this book, so chances are, you do not have this problem. However, sometimes the seventh chakra can shut down temporarily, in response to a spiritual crisis, depression, feelings of isolation, or a personal tragedy, such as the death of a loved one.

People with too-open seventh chakras relish the idea of a solitary life pursuing spiritual practices. They would do just fine living on mountaintops in the Himalayas or in monasteries or caves. In the real world, however, seventh chakras should be balanced, particularly with first chakras. This results in the ideal for life in the world: grounded in the now, but with a blissful sense of spiritual connectedness to all things in the universe.

Unspinning the Myths

Now that you know what chakras are, let's talk about what they *aren't*. Some people think the chakras are the solution to all their problems. Fix the chakra and fix your life. Not exactly. Chakras reflect what is going on in our bodies, minds, and spirits. They are a little bit like a mirror, or an instrument panel, so we can read ourselves better. But the chakras don't *cause* the problems. Life brings us problems, and the decisions we make and the attitudes we foster either solve problems or create more. Don't blame your first chakra if you are feeling ungrounded or your fourth chakra for being too trusting or your sixth chakra for that bad dream that came true. Your chakras just help you to understand yourself, so you can make choices that create your best life.

However, that being said, tuning in to and even healing the chakras can help urge your body, mind, feelings, and spiritual life back onto the right path. They go hand in hand with who you are, so if you work on the whole package at once, you will have quicker results. Ground yourself by healing your first chakra (you learn how in Chapter 7), but also by eating more protein, getting your finances in order, or calling or visiting home if you've been away for a while. Throughout this book, we talk about a lot of other ways to get yourself back in order when your chakras reveal that things are askew, but the point here is that your chakras are there for you to read. They are not the original cause of anything.

Another myth about the chakras is that they are a gateway to potentially dangerous *Kundalini* energy. Maybe you've heard rumors about the *Kundalini*, or serpent power, and how it can transform you in positive and negative ways. Actually, negative press about *Kundalini* is less a myth than a misunderstanding. We talk more about *Kundalini* energy in Chapter 3, but for now, rest easy knowing that your chakras are your protection against this intense energy surge, not a facilitator. When you are ready for *Kundalini* energy, your chakras open up and let it through. If you aren't ready, your chakras close like a valve. (There are some exceptions to this, when people purposefully open their chakras in order to release *Kundalini*, but again, we talk about that in more detail in Chapter 3.)

Finally, people sometimes misunderstand what each chakra represents. Just to clear the air right now, we will tell you that:

- The first chakra is not your animal side. You don't have to worry that tapping into this chakra will make you so instinct-based that you will be ruled by your basest instincts, resort to violence, or lose control of all your good sense. This chakra is grounding, not wild.

◆ The second chakra is not *only* the sex chakra. It is also about pleasure, passion, creativity, and everything you love to do. It is about moving and doing more than sexual obsession. Sexuality is just one small part of this chakra.

◆ The third chakra is not the "bad" chakra. Power can be a positive thing for building self-esteem, getting things done in the world, and knowing who you are. Reclaim your third chakra and don't be ashamed of it!

◆ The fourth chakra is not only about loving others. It is also about loving and *healing* yourself, so don't focus all that energy outside toward others. If you save energy for yourself, you'll be a much more open and giving person because you have the inner resources.

◆ The fifth chakra isn't just about communicating to the world. It is also about listening to the world communicate to you, and discerning the true parts. This is an important power, so don't underestimate the importance of this chakra. Your neck might be hurting for a very good reason. Are you facing the truth?

◆ The sixth chakra is not just associated with psychic powers, and while this can be part of this chakra, for most people this is irrelevant. The sixth chakra isn't there just so you can become a clairvoyant and have your own television show. The sixth chakra is about intuition and learning to listen to your own inner voice. It is an inward-turning chakra that can lead you to deep wisdom and the answers you desire.

◆ The seventh chakra isn't necessarily about God. You don't have to believe in any particular god to tap into the power of this chakra. Instead, it is your connection to the eternal, the universal, the life force, or a higher power, depending on who you are and what makes sense to you.

Taking the Wheel

We would like you to use this book as an instruction manual for operating your own chakras in a way that can make a difference in your life. You can learn to see them, measure them, understand them, and even change them. Their condition reflects who you are at any given moment, so it only makes sense that you should learn everything you can about them. Are you ready to take the wheel and start driving?

The Least You Need to Know

- ◆ Chakras are spinning centers of life force energy (sometimes called *prana* or *chi*) in the body. You have already felt them, perhaps while doing yoga, getting a massage, or during a session with an energy healer, such as a Reiki practitioner.

- ◆ There are seven major chakras located along the midline of the body, from the base of the spine to the crown of the head. Each chakra governs a different aspect of the self: grounding and safety, movement and sexuality, personal power, love, communication, intuition, and spiritual connection.

- ◆ Your chakras do not affect you. You affect your chakras.

- ◆ Learning how to read and manipulate your own chakras is a powerful tool for balancing, healing, and improving your life.

2

Chakra *Shakti:* The Power Tradition

In This Chapter

- ◆ How we know about the chakras
- ◆ Chakras and yoga
- ◆ Chakras and Buddhism
- ◆ Chakras and meditation
- ◆ How chakras fit into your personal practice

Chakras? Who ever thought of such a thing? And how did anyone ever figure out what and where they were? The concept of spinning energy centers in the body has an ancient feel, and indeed, the chakra concept has been around for many thousands of years. It is integral to many different branches of yoga, and ideas about chakras have evolved and changed (along with yoga itself) over the last 20 centuries or so. We promise not to bore you with a lot of history or technical detail, but let's take a brief look at how chakras originated, and what they mean in context. In this chapter, you not only find out why chakras have such clout, but also the ways you might be most comfortable thinking about and working with them.

Chakras' Origins: On the Wheels of Chariots

The first written texts in India are called the *Vedas*, a huge body of literature probably dating back as far as 2000 B.C.E. Before the *Vedas*, knowledge was passed along orally, and the *Vedas* probably include information that had been a part of Indian culture long before anyone thought to write down any of it. The *Vedas* are considered sacred texts in the Hindu religion, and they were written in *Sanskrit*, one of the ancient languages of India. The *Vedas* consist of several different works, including hymns, chants, stories, prophecies, and more. They are long, so unless you decide to become a Hindu scholar, you probably won't get around to reading them … even in translation! In orthodox Hinduism, however, the *Vedas* are sacred, considered passed down by God, and not something people just wrote down without any divine guidance.

The *Vedas* are the first place where the chakras are mentioned, and since, as we said, the *Vedas* are the oldest written text in India and among the oldest of written texts in the world, that means people have been talking about, thinking about, and writing about chakras for a lot longer than they have been talking, thinking, and writing about a lot of things.

According to chakra expert Anodea Judith, part of the *Vedas* contain the story of the Indo-European invasion when the Aryans stormed into India on wheeled chariots. The wheels of those chariots were described as *cakras*. The Aryans were also described as *cakravartins*, and the story says that golden wheels of light preceded their chariots. We can only speculate about what these golden disks of light might have been. Gold adornments to their chariots? Weapons? Judith wonders if it might have been the glow of their excessively powerful third chakras, which certainly would have had to be pretty fired up in order to conquer another race.

Judith also writes that the chakras were mentioned in the *Upanishads*—Hindu scriptures—around 600 C.E. They are also briefly mentioned in the *Yoga Sutras* written by the Hindu sage *Patanjali*, even though they are in no way central to that famous collection of aphorisms still often quoted today in yoga classes.

def•i•ni•tion

The **Upanishads** are Hindu scriptures sacred to the **Vedanta** branch of Hinduism. The **Yoga Sutras**, written by the Hindu sage **Patanjali**, are a collection of aphorisms defining yoga, written in the second century.

Chakras and Yoga: A Match Made in Heaven

Yoga is the practice of yoking together the body, mind, and spirit (to put it in very simple terms). Chakras are energy centers that also serve to link these different levels of the self, and the concept of chakras has been an integral part of yogic philosophy for thousands of years. However, not every branch of yoga emphasizes or even mentions chakras. The concept caught on and became a more central part of yoga with the development of *Tantra*.

Tantra is a branch of yoga that developed in the seventh century as a response to the previous notion (which many yogis still embrace) that we should rise above our physical lives, desires, and senses, to achieve a higher plane of existence. According to Tantra, our physical lives, desires, and senses are not bad things. In fact, they are real and worth embracing because they are the physical manifestation of divine energy. To live in the physical world and accept both its light and dark aspects is to worship God. This is also a central concept when working with chakras, as each chakra encompasses both the light and dark sides of the human body, mind, and spirit.

Tantra was widespread and took many forms, including *Kashmir Shavism*, a Shiva-worshipping form that originated in the eighth and ninth centuries and spawned the notion of *Kundalini* energy, which we talk about more in Chapter 5. *Kundalini* energy—the female aspect of the divine, or feminine energy—lies coiled around the first chakra like a sleeping serpent. As each chakra is energized, she rises up, piercing each one and progressing on toward the Crown chakra where she can finally unite with her beloved, the god Shiva, or the masculine principle of the divine. This can result in enlightenment, even if it only lasts for a little while. According to many sources, it can also result in mental problems and hallucinations for people who are not ready to experience the serpent power. (Don't worry. We talk you through this in Chapter 5.)

Kundalini energy rises like a serpent, energizing each chakra.

Westerners first heard about the chakras through a book published in 1919 called *The Serpent Power*, in which an Englishman named Arthur Avalon translated older *Hindu* texts and explained concepts like tantra, *kundalini*, and the chakras. This is only one of many interpretations, however. As any scholar versed in the subject will tell you, different schools of thought and various Hindu texts throughout history describe the chakras in many different ways. Some describe hundreds or even thousands of chakras. Some say there are eight chakras, or seven, or only five. Some say the chakras are energy centers, and others say they are regions in the body.

def·i·ni·tion

Hinduism is the predominant religion of India, where it began. Hindus have many diverse beliefs but many embrace the concepts of a supreme being and of reincarnation.

But this isn't a scholarly text, so we'll work to simplify as easily as we can and distill what we and others have learned about the chakras into information that will be useful to you in your daily life. (If you want more scholarly information, historical context, or anything else beyond the scope of this book, please see our resources section in Appendix B, to continue your study.)

Chakras and the Eightfold Path

We mostly think of chakras in terms of yoga, but remember that *Buddhism* began in India too, even though it is now more widespread in Asia. The idea of chakras isn't central to Buddhism, but the *Noble Eightfold Path* of Buddhism is often depicted as a spinning wheel with eight spokes that represent the eight aspects of the *Noble Eightfold Path*. (For more information about the Eightfold Path and other aspects of Buddhism, you might want to read *The Complete Idiot's Guide to Zen Living, Second Edition*, which Eve co-wrote with Gary McClain, Ph.D.)

def·i·ni·tion

Buddhism is a religion that began in India over 2,000 years ago with a man named Siddhartha Gautama, who became enlightened and is now known as the Buddha. Today millions of people all over the world practice several branches of Buddhism, although Buddhism is most widespread in Asia. The **Noble Eightfold Path** is the fourth of the Four Noble Truths of Buddhism. It consists of guidelines for living that help increase knowledge and maximize the chances for enlightenment. The eight paths are right understanding, right thought, right speech, right action, right livelihood, right effort, right mindfulness, and right concentration. The Noble Eightfold Path is often represented by a chakra called the *dharma wheel* or *dharmachakra* in Sanskrit. This is a symbol of a wheel with eight spokes representing each limb of the Noble Eightfold Path.

Because Hinduism and Buddhism both began in India, the Eightfold Path of Buddhism is probably related at its beginnings to the Eight Limbs of Yoga, which Patanjali wrote about in the *Yoga Sutras*. These aren't the same eight limbs as the limbs of the *Noble Eightfold Path*, but the idea is the same: to offer guidelines for living that will maximize physical and spiritual development.

The Eight Limbs of Yoga aren't directly related to the chakras, except that if you are practicing yoga, you should be aware of them since they are so essential to yogic thought. Unlike the Eightfold Path of Buddhism, the Eight Limbs of Yoga aren't typically depicted as a chakra, but practicing these eight limbs is energizing and balancing for all the chakras, so we go over them briefly:

- The *Yamas*, which are five positive practices to help you resist negative things like violence and lying. They are: *ahimsa*, non-violence; *satya*, telling the truth; *asteya*, not stealing; *brahmacharya*, abstaining from sexual misconduct; and *aparigraha*, not being jealous or coveting what others have. Practicing the *yamas* are particularly helpful for energizing the bottom four chakras.

- The *Niyamas*, which are five observances, or things to practice to enhance your life: *shaucha*, being pure by practicing cleanliness (in body and mind); *santosha*, being content or satisfied; *tapas*, being self-disciplined; *svadhyaya*, studying both the self and sacred texts; and *ishvarapranidhana*, worshipping God or surrendering to a Higher Power. Practicing the *niyamas* are particularly helpful for energizing the top three chakras.

- *Asana*, disciplining the body through yoga poses. Note that this is just one of the Eight Limbs of Yoga, even though many people today think of *asana* as the entirety of yoga. As you can see throughout this book, there are *asanas* that are particularly good for each chakra.

- *Pranayama*, or breath control through specific breathing exercises. *Pranayama* is good for all the chakras, depending on which type of breathing exercise you do, but particularly energizing for the fourth or Heart chakra.

- *Pratyahara*, the purposeful withdrawal of the senses for greater control over the mind. This is an excellent exercise for unblocking and energizing the sixth chakra.

- *Dharana*, or concentration, for mastery of the mind. This is particularly helpful for energizing and unblocking the sixth and seventh chakra.

- *Dhyana*, or meditation. Meditation is good for all the chakras, but particularly the province of the seventh chakra.

◆ *Samadhi*, or the experience of the unity of all things. When all your chakras are energized and awakened, you may have beautiful flashes of *Samadhi*.

Energy Unplugged _____

It's easy to take the concept of *ahimsa* literally: don't hurt or kill things. However, you can think of violence or harm in many ways, not just the physical. If you speak harshly to someone, or even think harsh thoughts about yourself, that is a form of violence. So is self-neglect. Also consider the ripple effect of your actions. Are you eating things that experienced violence so you could consume them? To some, vegetarianism is a crucial way to practice *ahimsa*, while to others, it is less important than, say, protesting war or working to stop domestic violence in their communities, or even being kind to themselves so they are able to then help and care for others. Think about what *ahimsa* means to you, and then you can move forward in your actions with confidence and conviction.

The Eight Limbs of Yoga aren't just similar to the Eightfold Path of Buddhism. They also sound a little bit like the Ten Commandments (for those of you who paid attention in your Sunday School classes). In other words, they are good advice and they promote physical, mental, and spiritual health. Those are all good for your chakras, so if you've been looking for some lifestyle guidance, there you have it!

Chakra Mind, Chakra Matters

Now that we are smack in the middle of the Age of Information, with the Internet facilitating instant transmission of knowledge from anywhere to anywhere else on the globe, millions of people know about chakras, yoga, Patanjali, Buddhism, Sanskrit, and all the other things we've talked about in this chapter. They don't all know how each of these things originated or what they mean in their historical context, but they know the words and many of us use those words often. We think about what they mean for us, in our twenty-first century lives. Considering the ancient history of these ideas, that's amazing.

Today, people use the concept of chakras in all sorts of contexts that they were never originally intended. But who says that's not okay? Chakras have followed us into the twenty-first century and still spin and open and close and work inside our bodies, so why shouldn't we adapt our thinking about them to match our lives? Of course we should.

One of the most common ways people work with chakras today is through *meditation* because the calm and stillness of mind you gain from meditation can help you tune in to how each chakra feels. Meditation techniques can also help you access your chakras in other ways, as you'll see throughout this book.

Meditation is defined in many ways by different people and traditions, and if you read about meditation, you can find numerous techniques, from slow counting or focusing on the breath to repeating a *mantra*, staring at and contemplating a *mandala*, considering illogical puzzles that push the mind beyond its logical limitations, or "just sitting" (*zazen*) to let all fluctuations of the mind dissipate, until it becomes like still water with no ripples.

Entering a labyrinth like this one from Chartres cathedral in France can be like entering spinning chakra energy, only to travel to rest at the divine center of being.

!!! **Wake-Up Call** _____

Meditation is a mental technique for quieting and focusing the mind, but it isn't as easy as it sounds. Sitting still and quieting the mind is incredibly challenging, and while it gets easier with practice, some people find it frustrating. In some cases, meditation is even counter-indicated. If you are feeling low on energy or depressed, you may get a more positive and helpful lift from exercise such as yoga poses rather than the inner-focusing work of meditation.

To some, meditation is good for stress relief, relaxation, or to work out problems and find solutions. To others, it is mental exercise, the brain's equivalent to the body's workout at the gym. To still others, the point is to experience only the present moment with no journeys to the past or future. Many use meditation as a form of prayer or communion with God, the divine spirit, or universal energy.

Meditation is also an integral part of the yogic path. The physical practice of yoga, the *asanas*, were developed to prepare the body for seated meditation. Meditation allows the mind to quiet and achieve such one-pointed concentration that you can perceive and actually experience the one-ness of all things. Yogic meditation is the path to ultimate unity with all living things, during which the person meditating understands that all is one.

This is also the goal of *Kundalini*, during her journey from the first chakra to the crown: to merge with Shiva in ultimate union, symbolizing the great unity of all life. Therefore, it makes logical sense that meditation and the chakras go together.

To begin meditating on your own chakras, sit quietly and tune in to each chakra, one at a time. Begin with the first chakra, at the base of the spine. Visualize its color, try to feel it spinning, and imagine what it looks like. Is it round? Crooked? Does it have any dents or dark spots? Is it in line with your spine? Which way is it turning? Imagine filling it with color and light to energize and balance it, then move on to the second chakra, just above the navel.

Proceed in the same way for the third chakra at the solar plexus, the fourth chakra at the heart, the fifth chakra in the throat, the sixth chakra in the forehead, and the seventh chakra at the crown of the head. Checking in each day with a meditative look at your own chakras can tell you a lot about what you need at any given moment: what your current strengths are, and where you need a little more loving care.

Meditate on the chakras.

Owning the Chakras

Remember that although many great scholars and wise people have written about the chakras throughout history, your chakras belong to you, right here, right now. That's the point of this book: not to school you on chakra philosophy, but to help you own your chakras, work with them, balance them, heal them, and become a better, more fully realized person because of that inner work.

Maybe you'll find the best way to work with your own chakras will be through the poses of Hatha yoga, or through mindful meditation, or through reading translations of some of the ancient sacred texts of yoga. Maybe you prefer the Tantric approach of embracing the physical world, or maybe you are more comfortable with a prayer-like communion with God to help balance your chakras.

Whatever way you choose to work with your chakras, this book can help you through it. If you love learning (your seventh chakra does!), the next chapter introduces you to chakra correspondences in the world. You learn how to tune in to the spinning wheels that make up our bodies, our cultures, and even our universe, from the atoms that comprise us to the solar systems that carry us through space. But if you want to get right down to working with your chakras, skip to Chapter 4, where we help you tune in to and even measure yours. Remember, they are your chakras, so forge your own path. We are right behind you.

The Least You Need to Know

♦ The first mention of chakras in written texts is in the *Vedas,* the oldest written texts of India. Chakras are also mentioned in the *Upanishads,* the *Yoga Sutras of Patanjali,* and many other ancient yoga and Hindu texts.

♦ A central concept in Buddhism is the Noble Eightfold Path, which offers guidelines for living. The Eightfold Path is typically depicted as a wheel with eight spokes called the dharma wheel or *dharmachakra.*

♦ In Patanjali's Yoga Sutras, he writes about the Eight Limbs of Yoga, which are similar guidelines for living. Although they are not depicted in wheel form, each limb is energizing and balancing for the chakras.

♦ Remember that your chakras are a tool for your own personal development, so as you work with them and explore them, choose the techniques that make the most sense for you.

Prana and Nadis and Chi ... Oh, My!

In This Chapter

◆ *Prana*, *chi*, *nadis*, meridians, and how they fit together

◆ The primary energy channels that influence the chakras and how to use them

◆ Easy *chi kung* to intensify your *chi*

Chakras are only a part of a complex esoteric Eastern view of the body your Western medical doctor never encountered during medical school. It's a different way of thinking about reality itself, and a product of a different culture than ours. But that doesn't mean it isn't worth consideration because the anatomical and spiritual view of the body so familiar to those growing up in India is not just well-established but time-honored and enduring in many other countries around the world. You already know this isn't a book about esoteric Indian health practices or Chinese medicine or Eastern theology. This is a book about you and the energy flow inside your own body. That means we are going to have to simplify things a bit. However, we don't want you to miss out on any of the good stuff, so in this chapter, we'll talk about the Indian view of anatomy, and what it means to you.

For now, we draw this picture in broad strokes, so you get all the information you need, without a lot of unnecessary extras. This chapter gives you the tools to understand your energy body and see what it's doing, so you can begin to understand how your chakras work in conjunction with everything else.

Get Prana

First, let's talk about what moves you. Or, more precisely, let's talk about the energy that flows through you. Let's talk about *prana*.

As we explained in Chapter 1, *prana* is the Sanskrit term for life force energy. Technically, there are several levels of *prana*, but for now, let's just talk about prana as the energy that flows in and out of the body and in and out of all living things. Sometimes, the word *prana* is used as a synonym for breath, but *prana* is not the same as breath. The breath is actually a vehicle to carry *prana* in and out of the body. *Prana* rides on and infuses the breath, but is not the breath.

def•i•ni•tion

Ayurveda is a traditional, holistic system of medicine that emphasizes a whole-life approach to health and life extension, including physical and breathing exercises, diet, massage, herbal medicine, and meditation.

Prana is a key element in *Ayurveda*, the ancient Indian science of health and longevity. According to Ayurveda, a body with free-flowing *prana* will be healthy. Blocks and overloads in the *prana* can lead to illness and disease. Ayurveda takes a holistic approach to health. By balancing *prana* through exercise, breathing, good hygiene, diet, massage, herbal medicine, and other specific practices, *prana* will become balanced and the body will heal itself, allowing the full expression of life: an integrated body, mind, and spirit.

This view of health and healing, along with the idea of *prana*, is an ancient one, and not unique to India. You might have heard about *chi* or *qi*, the word for life force energy that comes from China and is so often used in discussions of *acupuncture*, *Shiatsu massage*, *Traditional Chinese Medicine (TCM)*, and *Tai Chi Chuan* or *Chi Kung* (sometimes called *Qi Gong*).

Chi is essentially the same thing as *prana*. It is called *ki* in Japanese, *khi* in Vietnamese, and *gi* in Korean. They are the same words in different languages. These other systems of healing in other countries are, in essence, the same as Ayurveda. They all perceive that blocked, overloaded, or imbalanced life force energy leads to ill health and disease, while balanced, free-flowing energy leads to vibrant health and an integrated body, mind, and spirit. As opposed to Western medicine, which seeks to treat specific symptoms or physical abnormalities, these energy-based healing systems step back and see the body in a more holistic way. Correct the body's energy and the body will take care of the rest.

def•i•ni•tion

Acupuncture is a Chinese healing technique for freeing the flow of *chi* in the body by piercing energy centers with thin needles. Acupuncture relieves pain and promotes healing. **Shiatsu massage** is a Chinese healing technique in which the massage therapist uses manual pressure on acupressure points to correct energy imbalances. **TCM** is a system of healing techniques based on traditional Chinese health practices. These may include acupuncture, herbal and other remedies, and special exercises and massage designed to correct energy imbalances. **Tai Chi Chuan** is a form of Chinese martial arts related to **Chi Kung**, primarily practiced today as a meditative moving exercise to balance life force energy. Chi Kung, also called **Qi Gong**, is the art and practice of manipulating *chi* through movement and breath control.

Nadi or Nice?

Prana flows in and out of the body, but how? Just as water flows over the planet or electricity flows through a power plant, *prana* moves through the body via certain channels or meridians of energy. In Sanskrit, these channels are called *nadis*. In Chinese medicine, they are called meridians or channels. Again, however, the concept is basically the same.

Technically, *nadi* comes from the Sanskrit root *nad*, which means "movement." The word has been used in many ways in ancient yogic texts and Hindu scriptures. You could say that every blood vessel, artery, nerve, and breathing tube in your body is a *nadi* because *nadis* are basically passages through which something moves. In yoga, however, *nadis* generally refer specifically to the channels that carry life force energy, or *prana*.

Healers who are schooled in the subtleties of *nadis* or energy meridians use this knowledge in their practices. For example, according to Dr. Richard Gerber in his book *A Practical Guide to Vibrational Medicine*, knowing that, for example, a particular meridian passes through both the stomach and the knee joint can explain why people with knee arthritis or bursitis might also suffer from stomach problems. He writes, "It is not unusual for people to experience pain along a meridian pathway if there are physical problems affecting the corresponding meridian-linked organ."

For most of us, however, we don't have the time or resources to study every single meridian and its course through the body. We leave that to our healing professionals. Your body contains thousands of *nadis*, and it would take a long time and a lot of training to master them all. However, you can learn about three important ones that are directly related to your chakras. These are *nadis* you can influence through your own breathwork, movement, and even thought. They are *sushumna nadi*, *ida nadi*, and *pingala nadi*.

def•i•ni•tion

Sushumna nadi is a large central energy channel that runs along the spinal column from the base of the spine to the crown of the head. ***Ida nadi*** is the energy channel that carries feminine energy from the base of the spine to the left of *sushumna nadi*, coiling around the spine in opposition to ***pingala nadi***, and ending at the left nostril. *Pingala nadi* is the energy channel that carries masculine energy from the base of the spine to the right of *sushumna nadi*, coiling around the spine in opposition to *ida nadi*, and ending at right nostril.

Sushumna Nadi

One of the most important *nadis* in your body is *sushumna nadi*. This is the central *nadi* that runs along the midline of your body, right along your spinal column. It isn't your spinal column, but it coincides with your spinal column.

Sushumna begins at your first chakra and ends at your seventh chakra, piercing the center of each chakra. Somewhere around the sixth chakra, behind your forehead, the *sushumna nadi* divides into two, like a fork in the road. The front side moves straight up to the seventh chakra at the crown of the head. The back side curves around the back side of your brain and meets the front side at the seventh chakra.

Sushumna nadi is important because this is the channel that carries *Kundalini* energy from the base of the spine to the crown of the head. In his book *Light on Pranayama*, B.K.S. Iyengar writes: "Through the discipline of yoga, the direction of the mouth of the coiled serpentine energy is made to turn upwards. It rises like steam through the sushumna ... till it reaches the sahasrara." That serpentine energy is *Kundalini*. We talk more about that in Chapter 4, but for now, just remember that *sushumna nadi* is *Kundalini's* private highway.

In order to ascend through the *sushumna nadi*, *Kundalini* must move through each of the primary seven chakras along the spine. In order for that to happen, those chakras have to be open, healthy, and free-flowing.

Ida and *Pingala Nadis*

Wrapped around *sushumna* are two other important *nadis* that cross and recross each other at each chakra. These are the *ida* and *pingala nadis. Ida* and *pingala nadis* begin at the base of the spine, to the left and right (respectively) of *sushumna nadi.* (Some texts say they begin higher up, around the second chakra.) *Ida* and *pingala* coil around *sushumna nadi* in a sort of double-helix pattern, intertwining and crossing each other at each chakra point. Some people compare this structure to a strand of DNA, or to the Greek *caduceus* symbol of two snakes entwined around a staff. Indeed, the staff is like *sushumna nadi* and the two snakes are like *ida* and *pingala*, so this is an appropriate way to think about it.

The caduceus symbol.

def•i•ni•tion

The **caduceus** is a Greek symbol used today to represent the practice of medicine. It depicts a staff with two snakes entwining around it from bottom to top. This symbol is often used to describe the way in which the masculine and feminine energy channels or *nadis* coil around a central energy channel in the body, called *sushumna nadi,* which runs along the spinal column.

Like the Chinese concept of *yin* and *yang* energy, *ida* and *pingala* each carry a different kind of energy. *Ida* transports lunar, female energy. It is a calm, cooling, meditative, receptive, centered energy that is good to channel during meditation. *Pingala* energy is active, energetic, heating, forceful energy that is good to channel when you need to get things done. When you breathe out of your left nostril, you tap into *ida's* energy. When you breathe out of the right nostril, you channel *pingala* energy.

Ida carries yin energy.
Pingala carries yang energy.

According to yogic belief, we all tend to breathe primarily out of one nostril at certain times during the day, then out of the other. Depending on which nostril is dominant at any given moment, that is the energy that is flowing, either through *ida* or *pingala*. For a few breaths each hour, when our breath is shifting from one nostril to the other, we breathe out of both nostrils at the same time, activating the *sushumna nadi*.

def•i•ni•tion

Yin and yang are terms for opposite but balancing forces, according to ancient Chinese philosophy. All things have yin and yang energy. Yin energy is lunar, feminine, cooling, receptive energy. Yang energy is solar, masculine, heating, forceful energy. Yin energy is equivalent to the energy that moves through *ida nadi*. Yang energy is equivalent to the energy that moves through *pingala nadi*.

Pranayama exercises, which are meant to train and channel the breath to infuse our bodies with *prana*, can also influence the channels we use. In particular, *nadi shodhana*, or alternate nostril breathing, helps balance our *prana* along both *ida* and *pingala* by purposefully inhaling through one nostril while holding the other closed, then switching nostrils and exhaling out of the opposite nostril, then inhaling and switching again.

Ida and *pingala* are important to understand when working with the chakras because they can be helpful, depending on which chakra you are working on and whether that chakra is blocked or overloaded. *Ida* energy can help calm and dissipate an overloaded chakra, while *pingala* energy can help energize and open a blocked chakra. *Ida* energy is good for meditation, while *pingala* energy is good for invigorating exercise. Learn how to use these energies to your own benefit and you'll have another powerful tool for working with your chakras.

Chakras: Traffic Circles, Energy Transformers, Cosmic Vortices ... Pick a Metaphor

Now, imagine energy, or *prana*, flowing through your body, coursing through thousands of channels like a network of rivers and streams running through every inch from torso to fingertips, from the bottoms of your toes to the top of your head. *Nadis* run up and down your body, not just *sushumna*, *ida*, and *pingala*, but a lot of smaller ones, connecting, for example, your left ear to your right big toe (that one is called *yashasvini*) and your right ear to your left big toe (that one is called *pusha*). You've got *nadis* connecting your eyes to your feet, your throat to your genitals, your hands to your heart. You've got thousands of *nadis* splitting into thousands more smaller *nadis*, and all of them are filled with energy, moving and flowing. This is a road map of you.

Imagine those spots in this vast system of energy flow that are like whirlpools or vortices of energy, where big groups of rivers and streams come together into a swirling central area, then flow back out to other rivers and streams. They collect along your spine, in the palms of your hands, in the soles of your feet. These are your chakras.

If you read a lot about chakras, you read a lot of metaphors. Call them whirlpools in your network of rivers and streams, traffic circles on the interstate highway system that is you, energy transformers in the vast power plant of your body, or cosmic vortices in your individual manifestation of universal energy. What you call them doesn't matter so much as how you use them.

Because chakras are energy centers where *prana* collects as it travels through the *nadis* of your body, these are energy-intensive spots with a lot of power. That power is yours, swirling there inside for you to read, feel, contemplate, and *use*. This energy belongs to you. In fact, it *is* you. So you might as well start tapping into it.

Tuning Up the System

Now that you have a general idea of the network of energy running through your body, we would like you to start feeling it.

Of course, you already feel your own energy flow all the time, as you go through your daily life. Whenever you get a surge of energy or good feeling, and also when you feel blocked or low on energy or depressed, you are perceiving your own energy flow. Excitement, fright, anxiety, nervousness, contentment, all these reflect what your energy is doing at any given moment. However, feeling your energy and really focusing in on your energy are two different things.

Feel the energy of your Heart chakra.

Any physical exercise can help get *prana* or *chi* moving in your body, but *Chi Kung*, the art and practice of manipulating *chi* in the body, consists of different exercises that specifically move and intensify your inner *chi*. The exercise below is particularly good for drawing in and strengthening inner *chi*. In fact, some say that with the regular practice of this exercise, you can build such inner strength that you can break a board without ever doing any other muscle-strengthening exercises.

Chi Kung Windmill

This exercise is adapted from an exercise that Gene Wong taught to David Carradine, as described in his book *Introduction to Chi Kung*.

- ◆ Stand with your feet a little wider than shoulder-width apart and your toes pointed forward. Settle your weight into your heels and bend your knees just slightly, but not so much that they extend past the feet. Tuck your tailbone in, pull your chin slightly in, and lift up at the crown of your head. broaden your upper and middle back and imagine sending energy forward from the area just over your navel. This is the appropriate stance for many *chi kung* exercises.

- ◆ Hold your left palm facing up against your abdomen. Raise your right hand in front of you, palm facing out, and look at the back of your hand. Slowly and with control, move your palm up, keeping your elbow slightly bent. Move your arm in a big circle, like a windmill blade, back behind you and around, following the back of your hand with your eyes.

- ◆ Bring your right hand, palm up, against your abdomen and rotate your left arm in a big circle, following the back of your hand with your eyes.

- ◆ Repeat several times with both arms.

Do this exercise every day and enjoy dramatic energy reserves. This exercise is also particularly energizing for the third chakra.

Now that we've got those chakras into perspective, let's explore them in more depth. Circles, after all, penetrate our culture, our biology, our universe. Keep reading to find out how.

The Least You Need to Know

- Life force energy that moves in and out of the body with the breath is called *prana* in Sanskrit, *chi* in Chinese, *ki* in Japanese, and other things in other languages, but these all refer to basically the same energetic force.

- *Nadis*, meridians, or channels are all terms used to describe the passageways for energy throughout the body. Practitioners of Ayurveda, acupuncture, Shiatsu massage, *Chi Kung*, and many other disciplines use these meridians to free the flow of life force energy for healing and longevity.

- Chakras are the vortices or centers of energy along the meridians in the body.

- Simple *Chi Kung* exercises get *chi* moving and can strengthen inner power.

Part 2

Dynamics of Chakra Force

Chakra means wheel, and this part of the book gets into more depth about how those inner wheels actually work: how they turn, how they manipulate and dispense energy, and exactly what they do. We explore the notorious *Kundalini* energy that lies coiled around your first chakra, waiting to be awakened. We talk about myths and truths associated with *Kundalini*, and how you can energize yours. Finally, we show you how to tune in to your chakras, measure them, and diagnose your own chakra blockages and overloads, for better health, mental clarity, emotional balance, and who knows … maybe even spiritual enlightenment.

Chapter 4

Going 'Round in Circles

In This Chapter

- ◆ The many kinds of wheels in the physical universe
- ◆ The inner workings of the chakras
- ◆ Understanding blocks and overloads

From an atom to a galaxy, the physical world is filled with spinning wheels. Chakras, those spinning wheels of life force energy within us, may not be visible with medical imaging equipment, but they mirror the physical world in its countless manifestations of the same shape and movement. The wheel, circle, spiral, vortex—the concept is practically a motif for physical reality. In this chapter, we explore what it means to be going around in circles.

Wheels of Life

Think about an atom, the smallest possible piece of something that still has the chemical properties of that thing. Atoms make up all matter in the universe. You can't see them because light particles are too large to illuminate them. Traditionally, atoms have always been depicted as a central nucleus made of protons and neutrons surrounded by orbiting electrons.

Now, scientists think that the electrons around an atom's nucleus are probably moving more randomly, in a cloud around the nucleus; but nevertheless, the shape is probably round, with particles surrounding a center.

Chakras are spinning energy.

But let's get bigger. Nature is filled with circles, spirals, and wheels, which chakras resemble. Look at the center of a flower, its petals curling around the bud. Consider the shape of a raindrop as it splashes onto the pavement, or the ripples that move out over the surface of a pond when you skip a stone across the surface. Look into the eyes of a person, an animal, even an insect, see the circles within circles. Our finger-prints contain circles and spirals. So do snail shells and ….

Let's think even bigger. Tornadoes, hurricanes, waterspouts, and whirlpools all move in circles and spin like wheels. Planets, moons, and suns are spheres with moons moving around planets and planets moving around suns. Entire galaxies full of millions of stars and solar systems move in circles around a center.

Back on Earth, humans like to make circles, too. Not only did we invent the wheel, but we also invented clocks, compasses, rings, crowns, cymbals, hula hoops, door-knobs, plates and saucers, Frisbees, and fans, not to mention computer hard drives that spin and store information much like a chakra does. We have circles of friends and spheres of influence. We hold sewing circles and prayer circles. We use circles to unpuzzle geometry problems, and we engage in circular reasoning. Our culture has ideas about flying saucers and crop circles and ancient circular formations such as Stonehenge. We judge artistic skill by the ability to draw a perfect circle.

Our blood circulates through our bodies, air circulates through our lungs, and our heads spin with thoughts and feelings. It's no wonder our chakras spin, too. The more we reflect on circles and wheels as they are a part of human existence in the universe, the more it makes perfect sense that our energy flows through us and collects in powerful circles of energy.

Chakra Symbolism

Our culture is full of circle and wheel symbols, but each chakra also has its own slew of associations. Depending on what book you pick up, what website you surf, or who you hear expounding on the chakras, you can find lists not just of colors, body systems, and elements associated with the chakras, but also of planets, hand positions, numbers, zodiac signs, sections of the palms of the hands, key words, and types of people. Each chakra also has a seed sound which, when chanted, is thought to awaken that chakra. Each of these associations might suggest new ways of looking at and working with your own chakras. Here are just a few of the many chakra associations we've uncovered through our own research.

First Chakra

The first chakra, also called the Root chakra or *Muludhara*, has also been associated with the following:

- **Animal:** Snake, elephant, bull, ox
- **Archangel:** Auriel or Michael
- **Body:** Physical
- **Color:** Red
- **Element:** Earth
- **Food:** All food, but especially proteins like meat
- **Gemstone or crystal:** Ruby, cinnabar, bloodstone, garnet, or other red stones
- **Gods and Goddesses:** Atlas, Brahma, Demeter and Persephone, Gaia, Ganesha

Gaia holds first chakra energy.

- **Herbs/spices:** Ashwangandha
- **Incense:** Cedar
- **Keyword:** Security
- **Kinds of people:** Family members, including ancestors
- **Metal:** Lead
- **Musical note:** C
- **Number of lotus petals:** Four
- **Plane of existence:** Physical or material plane
- **Ruling planet:** Mars, Saturn, Earth
- **Seed sound:** LANG
- **Sense organ:** Nose
- **Sense:** Smell
- **Shape:** Square
- **Tarot suit:** Pentacles
- **Verb:** To have
- **Vowel or vibration:** U (as in "you") or OH (as in "rope")
- **Yoga path:** *Hatha yoga*
- **Zodiac signs:** Gemini and Cancer

Second Chakra

The second chakra, also called *Svadhisthana*, has been associated with the following:

- **Animal:** Fish and other sea creatures
- **Archangel:** Gabriel or Metatron
- **Body:** Emotional
- **Color:** Orange
- **Element:** Water
- **Food:** Sweet fruit such as melons, strawberries, mangoes, and coconut; honey; nuts; spices such as vanilla, carob, and cinnamon
- **Gemstone or crystal:** Carnelian, coral, amber, or other orange stones
- **Gods and Goddesses:** Diana, Dionysius, Indra, Pan, Rakini, Varuna, Vishnu
- **Herbs/spices:** Coriander, fennel
- **Incense:** Gardenia
- **Keyword:** Feeling
- **Kinds of people:** Children, romantic partners
- **Metal:** Tin
- **Musical note:** D
- **Number of lotus petals:** Six
- **Plane of existence:** Astral plane
- **Ruling planet:** Mercury, Jupiter, or the Moon
- **Seed sound:** VANG
- **Sense organ:** Tongue
- **Sense:** Taste
- **Shape:** Teardrop
- **Tarot suit:** Cups
- **Verb:** To feel
- **Vowel or vibration:** OH (as in "home") or OO (as in "due")

♦ **Yoga path:** Tantra yoga

♦ **Zodiac sign:** Taurus and Leo

Spinning Your Wheels _____

People often wonder why things like Tarot suits, Zodiac signs, or musical notes relate to each chakra. Actually, different traditions and even different individuals have different interpretations about what corresponds to each chakra. However, most of the correspondences are based not just in someone's intuition but in thousands of years of study of ancient texts, spiritual contemplation, and plain old similarity. People have likened the placement and spin of the chakras to many other aspects of human knowledge and consciousness, from the placement and spin of planets, the symbolism associated with Tarot cards, and the traditional aspects of life governed by various gods and goddesses, to a more scientific analysis of sound waves and light spectrums. In this chapter, we've listed some of the associations familiar to us, but there are others out there, and you might discover still more useful associations using your own intuition about your own chakras. That's all part of the fun!

Third Chakra

The third chakra, also called *Manipura*, has been associated with the following:

♦ **Animal:** Birds, the ram

♦ **Archangel:** Michael or Uriel

♦ **Body:** Mental

♦ **Color:** Yellow

♦ **Element:** Fire

♦ **Food:** Grains such as pasta, bread, rice, and cereal; seeds such as sunflower seeds, sesame seeds, and flax seeds; dairy products such as milk, cheese, and yogurt; mint; spices such as turmeric, ginger, and cumin

♦ **Gemstone or crystal:** Amber, topaz, citrine, gold, or other yellow or gold stones

♦ **Gods and Goddesses:** Agni, Athena, Helios, Lakini, Rudra, Surya

♦ **Herbs/spices:** Goldenseal, lemon balm

♦ **Incense:** Cinnamon, Dragon's blood, ginger

♦ **Keyword:** Opinion

- **Kinds of people:** Friends, colleagues
- **Metal:** Iron
- **Musical note:** E
- **Number of lotus petals:** Ten
- **Plane of existence:** Celestial plane
- **Ruling planet:** Sun or Mars
- **Seed sound:** RANG
- **Sense organ:** Eyes
- **Sense:** Sight
- **Shape:** Downward-pointing triangle
- **Tarot suit:** Wands
- **Verb:** To do
- **Vowel or vibration:** O (as in "top") or AH (as in "father")
- **Yoga path:** *Power yoga*
- **Zodiac sign:** Aries and Virgo

def•i•ni•tion

Power yoga is a contemporary form of yoga that combines traditional poses with challenging and dynamic movements for a more intense physical workout.

Fourth Chakra

The fourth chakra, also called *Anahata,* has been associated with the following:

- **Animal:** Antelopes, doves, mammals with four legs
- **Archangel:** Raphael or Chamuel
- **Body:** Astral
- **Color:** Green
- **Element:** Air
- **Food:** Leafy green vegetables like kale, spinach, and lettuce; broccoli; celery; cabbage; squash; greens

- **Herbs/spices:** Basil, thyme, cilantro, and parsley; green tea

- **Gemstone or crystal:** Emerald, jade, malachite, green tourmaline, or other green stones

- **Gods and Goddesses:** Aphrodite, Eros, Jesus Christ, Krishna, Lakshmi

- **Herbs/spices:** Rue, saffron

- **Incense:** Lavender, jasmine

- **Keyword:** Love

- **Kinds of people:** Teachers, boddhisatvas (people who delay their own enlightenment to help others reach enlightenment)

- **Metal:** Copper

- **Musical note:** F

- **Number of lotus petals:** Twelve

- **Plane of existence:** Balance plane

- **Ruling planet:** Venus

- **Seed sound:** YANG

- **Sense organ:** Skin

- **Sense:** Touch

- **Shape:** Hexagram

- **Tarot suit:** Swords

- **Verb:** To love

- **Vowel sound:** AH (as in "far") or AY (as in "play")

- **Yoga path:** *Bhakti yoga*

- **Zodiac sign:** Pisces and Libra

def•i•ni•tion

Bhakti yoga is the yoga of devotion, involving the practice and expression of the emotional connection with God, universal spirit, or ultimate reality through chanting and worship rituals.

Fifth Chakra

The fifth chakra, also called *Vishuddha*, has been associated with the following:

- **Animal:** Humans, elephants, bulls, lions

- **Archangel:** Michael or Gabriel

- **Body:** Etheric

- **Color:** Blue

- **Element:** Ether or space

- **Food:** Fruit (especially tart fruits like citrus), fruit juice, herbal tea, salt

- **Gemstone or crystal:** Sapphire, lapis lazuli, turquoise, blue sapphire, sodalite, aquamarine, abalone, or other blue stones

- **Gods and Goddesses:** Apollo, Brigit, Ganga (the river goddess), Sarasvati

Sarasvati holds fifth chakra energy.

- **Herbs/spices:** Cloves, Vervain

- **Incense:** Frankincense, mace

- **Keyword:** Expression

- **Kinds of people:** Teachers and leaders

- **Metal:** Mercury

- **Musical note:** G

- **Number of lotus petals:** Sixteen

- **Plane of existence:** Human

- **Ruling planet:** Jupiter or Mercury

- **Seed sound:** HANG

- **Sense organ:** Ears

◆ **Sense:** Hearing

◆ **Shape:** Crescent

◆ **Tarot suit:** Wands

◆ **Verb:** To speak

◆ **Vowel sound:** EH (as in "let") or EE (as in "seen")

◆ **Yoga path:** *Mantra yoga*

◆ **Zodiac sign:** Aquarius and Scorpio

def•i•ni•tion

Mantra yoga is the practice of chanting a *mantra*, a sacred syllable or phrase that is spoken repeatedly to aid in concentration and focus.

Sixth Chakra

The sixth chakra, also called *Ajna*, has been associated with the following:

◆ **Animal:** *Archetypes*, owls

def•i•ni•tion

Archetypes, as first defined by psychologist Carl Jung, are powerful inner patterns or universal roles seen in all cultures, such as the villain, the hero, the maiden, the crone, the wise man, or the mother. These patterns of behavior unconsciously influence people's thoughts and actions relating to themselves and others, and have endured through much of human history, often played out in the mythologies of different cultures. For instance, many cultures have a "savior," a "virgin mother," and a "devil" of some kind.

◆ **Archangel:** Raphael

◆ **Body:** Celestial

◆ **Color:** Deep indigo or purple

◆ **Element:** Supreme element, a combination of all the other elements.

◆ **Food:** Blackberries, blueberries, purple grapes, poppy seeds, any food/substance that affects perception and intuition, including red wine

◆ **Gemstone or crystal:** Amethyst, alexandrite, azurite, fluorite, star sapphire, or other deep blue or purple stones

◆ **Gods and Goddesses:** Apollo, Hecate, Isis, Krishna, Paramasiva (form of Shiva), Shakti Hakini

- **Herbs/spices:** Sandalwood
- **Incense:** Star anise, acacia
- **Keyword:** Insight
- **Kinds of people:** Spiritual friends, the people it seems like you've "always known"
- **Metal:** Silver
- **Musical note:** A
- **Number of lotus petals:** Two
- **Plane of existence:** Austerity
- **Ruling planet:** Saturn or the Sun
- **Seed sound:** AUM
- **Sense organ:** Third eye
- **Sense:** Intuition
- **Shape:** A circle with two petals
- **Tarot suit:** Swords
- **Verb:** to see
- **Vowel or vibration:** EE (as in "me") or MM
- **Yoga path:** *Yantra yoga*
- **Zodiac sign:** Capricorn and Sagittarius

def•i•ni•tion

Yantra yoga is a Tibetan form of yoga similar to Hatha yoga that combines poses with breathing exercises and meditation to increase life force energy.

Seventh Chakra

The seventh chakra, also called *Sahasrara*, has been associated with the following:

- **Animal:** Spirits of the deceased, especially ancestral spirits
- **Archangel:** Jophiel
- **Body:** Causal or auric
- **Color:** Purple or white

- **Element:** Thought or God

- **Food:** None (fasting), or dark blue grapes, blackberries, garlic

- **Gemstone or crystal:** Diamond, amethyst, quartz crystal

- **Gods and Goddesses:** Allah, Ama-kala, Inanna, Nut, Odin, Shiva, Varuna

Inanna holds seventh chakra energy.

- **Herbs/spices:** Gotu kola, nutmeg

- **Incense:** Lotus, gotu kola

- **Keyword:** Freedom

- **Kinds of people:** Saints, prophets, true gurus

- **Metal:** gold

- **Musical note:** B

- **Number of lotus petals:** One thousand

- **Plane of existence:** Reality

- **Ruling planet:** Ketu, the southern point where the moon and the sun cross paths, or Uranus

- **Seed sound:** Universal vibration making the sound of AUM

- **Sense organ:** Brain

- **Sense:** Perception of God

- **Shape:** Circle

- **Tarot suit:** The entire Major Arcana (the 22 dominant Tarot cards in a standard deck)

- **Verb:** To know

- **Vowel or vibration:** AUM or OM (as in "ah-oo-oh-m") or Ngngng (as in "sing")

- **Yoga path:** *Jnana yoga*

- **Zodiac sign:** None

def•i•ni•tion

Jnana yoga is the yoga of knowledge, which is practiced by meditating on the self and studying spiritual texts.

Inside the Chakras

Each chakra has plenty of symbols and associations, but what's going on inside those inner energy circles we call the chakras? In the last chapter, we explained how life force energy moves in and out and through the body via meridians or channels, called *nadis* in yoga. Inside the chakras, energy also moves in and out, in a lot of different ways, depending on what's going on with you.

If you could see your own chakras (which some people can, through meditation techniques), you might see clear colored wheels of energy turning clockwise. Or, you might see some disturbances. A lot of things can happen to a chakra from moment to moment. Our chakras change size, shape, and speed of spin throughout the day. They are taking in *prana*, processing it so the body can use it, and releasing it back into the system, like energy transformers.

However, sometimes things go awry. A temporary change in a chakra isn't a big deal, but chronic changes can indicate a problem. Chakras don't cause problems, they reflect problems in your body, mind, or spirit. In Chapter 6, we show you how to measure your own chakras and give you the opportunity to feel your own chakras through a simple exercise. In Chapter 19, we walk you through a meditative exercise to help you see your own chakras, but for now, let's talk about what they are doing, whether you can see them or not.

Healthy Chakras

Healthy chakras are the ideal, and chances are, most of your chakras are doing pretty well most of the time. A healthy chakra takes in *prana*, spins it around, and shoots it out again. Healthy chakras appear round, with solid borders, bright color, and a clock-wise spin.

*The spinning energy of a
healthy third chakra.*

Before we move on to working with your chakras, we have one more interesting aspect of the chakra system to cover: the mysterious, notorious, and much-misunderstood *Kundalini*. Check out the next chapter to learn more about your own personal serpent power.

The Least You Need to Know

◆ Our bodies, our culture, our world, and our universe are full of circle and wheel symbols, from the smallest atom to the largest galaxy.

◆ Each of the seven major chakras has been associated with many different things, from colors and animals to zodiac signs, tarot suits, and certain kinds of foods.

◆ The chakras take in *prana*, process it for use by the body, and release it back into the *nadis*. Sometimes, chakras reflect imbalances in the body, mind, or spirit.

Kundalini: Be a Snake Charmer

In This Chapter

- What is *Kundalini*, and should you be afraid of it?

- Preparing the body for *Kundalini* rising

- How *Kundalini* moves through the chakras

- The transformative power of *Kundalini* energy

- How to awaken, move, and manipulate *Kundalini*

Perhaps no yoga concept is more misunderstood, feared, maligned, and sought-after than the concept of *Kundalini*. Yet no book about the chakras could be complete without it because *Kundalini* is an integral part of the entire chakra system. *Kundalini* has been discussed, debated, analyzed, and experienced by people practicing and studying yoga for thousands of years, but the secrets of *Kundalini* were always passed from guru to student orally. The student had to prove purity and discipline before learning the secrets. That is, until Yogi Bhajan, a *Kundalini* master, came to the United States and began to lecture publicly about *Kundalini*, beginning in 1969.

Since then, *Kundalini yoga* has become a widely practiced form of yoga, emphasizing awareness and the mobilization of the life force. Yogi Bhajan once said, famously, "If flexibility of the body is the only yoga, then clowns in the circus are the best yogis." In other words, *Kundalini* yoga (indeed, all true yoga) is much more than poses or *asanas*. In many traditions, that "much more" part has a lot to do with *Kundalini*.

As with any esoteric yoga concept that has been around for a while, different ancient and modern scholarly and popular texts discuss *Kundalini* in many different ways. Some directly contradict each other, and some are so steeped in the culture of India that they can be difficult for Westerners to comprehend. In this chapter, however, we're going to minimize the esoteric part and get right down to what you really want to know: what is your own *Kundalini* energy all about, and how can you make it work for you?

What *Kundalini* Is

Kundalini is an inner source of power that lives inside you. The word literally means "coiled," and *Kundalini* is often described as a coiled serpent lying at the base of your spine, within your first chakra. But if snakes freak you out, you don't have to think of *Kundalini* in this way. *Kundalini* isn't some foreign presence in your body. It is part of you.

def•i•ni•tion

Kundalini is a Sanskrit term meaning (approximately) "coiled one." *Kundalini* is also an ancient, esoteric yoga concept that feminine energy lies coiled like a serpent at the base of the spine inside the first chakra. As *Kundalini* energy is awakened through spiritual practices like yoga, she desires to merge with masculine energy (sometimes represented as the Hindu god Shiva) so she rises up through each chakra as it opens, energizing and activating that chakra. The result is gradual awakening leading to enlightenment, and the intense activation of creative energy and spiritual awareness in the body. *Kundalini* yoga is a form of yoga that seeks to awaken and utilize *Kundalini* energy through poses, meditation, chanting, breathing exercises, and other techniques, with the ultimate goal of realizing the individual's inner divinity and oneness with God and all creation.

Kundalini is divine power within you, which is separate from (and incomplete without) the divine power of the universe. *Kundalini* yoga seeks to join the two, so that you can realize and truly comprehend your own inner divinity and your connection with God, universal energy, or whatever the external sacred force of life is to you.

Kundalini *lays coiled at the base of the spine.*

When these two are yoked together—your own divinity and universal divinity—through *Kundalini*-arousing techniques, you reach a new level of understanding, a sort of spiritual evolutionary leap forward. It isn't necessarily a permanent leap, but more often a glimpse of or a temporary immersion into your highest self.

Energy Unplugged

Can you perceive, believe in, and awaken *Kundalini* without believing in any particular God? What if you aren't sure about the whole "Higher Power" concept at all? No problem. *Kundalini* is the source of divinity within you. It is yours, and it is the catalyst for connecting to all of life. But that can mean different things to different people. We can describe *Kundalini* only in mere words, which pale in comparison to the actual experience of it. This is about a universal quest for meaning, so rather than abandoning that quest over semantics, let that quest take you in a direction that makes sense for you.

Because *Kundalini* is a difficult concept to grasp, people often explain it using metaphors. One of the most common is that *Kundalini* is a goddess who seeks her male counterpart, Shiva. When aroused, she rises up through the chakras to reach Shiva at the crown chakra, where they merge in holy union. Remember, this is a metaphor, and one that makes sense to people in India who are familiar with Shiva and the idea of other gods and goddesses.

But this metaphor might not work so well for you. After all, your spinal column isn't a celestial hook-up spot. The idea of a union between *Kundalini* and Shiva simply represents the union of your consciousness with universal consciousness. It is a glimpse into the divine spark within you. To put it in more Western terms, *Kundalini* rising is like experiencing your own perfection by finally seeing your place in the universal scheme of things. This is the answer to "Who am I and what does it all mean?" When *Kundalini* reaches your seventh chakra, you know the answer to that question.

In Kama Sutra, this position arouses Kundalini and is called Shakti Expressing Her Energy with Shiva.

No, we can't just tell you the answer to save time. Each individual person is a unique manifestation of divine energy. You are the only *you* in the universe, and when you recognize yourself at last, that recognition will be entirely unique. According to yoga philosophy, we are all one, and one with the divine universal presence, but at the same time, we are all different, too. During our time on Earth, in these bodies we live in for a little while, we perceive our immense diversity. And yet, we also have the capacity to understand our ultimate unity. Pretty cool, right?

But it isn't easy. You can't just kick *Kundalini* awake and sit back waiting for the ecstasy to start rolling in. Awakening *Kundalini* for ultimate universal fusion takes time, preparation, and commitment (like any good relationship). *Kundalini* is one of the gifts we get in this life, along with our bodies, minds, and spirits. We can waste it, or we can use it to become better, happier, clearer, healthier, and more at peace.

What *Kundalini* Isn't

You might be wondering about some of the things you've heard about *Kundalini*. If you read about *Kundalini*, you may run across references to the dangers of prematurely awakening the "serpent power." Maybe you've read that when *Kundalini* moves, you can experience weird bodily sensations like intense heat or cold in the spinal column, feelings of fluttering or slithering, spontaneous movements of your body, even hearing voices or hallucinating. We've even read about violent reactions to *Kundalini* awakenings, complete psychotic breaks, and death. That sounds pretty scary, doesn't it?

Okay, you can stop worrying now. There are quite a lot of theories about the so-called dangers of awakening *Kundalini,* but the simple truth is that *Kundalini* is part of you, and inner awakening doesn't hurt you. In many cases, people who have violent psychopathic episodes associated with supposed *Kundalini* awakenings already suffer from mental illness.

In other cases, people were so immersed in hours and hours of meditation that they threw themselves out of balance. When accompanied by fasting (on purpose or just because someone forgets to eat), the problem can be compounded through dehydration. Humans have incredibly complex minds and are susceptible to suggestion. Emotional and mental problems are fairly common in the human species, and sometimes these go hand in hand with the quest for religious experience or understanding of the self.

!!!) Wake-Up Call _____

If you have emotional or mental problems, intense immersion into the quest for awakening *Kundalini* could result in some psychological issues, but it isn't the *Kundalini* doing it. It is an imbalance within you, and that means you need to seek help from a professional who understands the context of your problems. We urge you to seek help from a counselor or therapist if you are suffering from an imbalance.

If you have physical, emotional, mental, or spiritual issues, *your chakras won't be healthy, balanced, and open.* And that means *Kundalini* won't rise. This is your body's own internal security system. If, on the other hand, you are a sound, healthy person who is balanced and primed for a spiritual experience, you are ready for *Kundalini* to rise. You aren't going to suffer a mental breakdown or drop dead because you practiced the *Kundalini*-awakening exercises in this book. We promise. When you are in an unhealthy state and you have a physical or emotional issue or episode, *it is not Kundalini.* It is something that needs to be addressed by a medical or mental health professional.

Kundalini is a powerful internal force, for sure, but it's *your* power. To repeat: if your chakras aren't open and ready (meaning you are not open and ready), *Kundalini* can't move up through them. They will keep *Kundalini* down by closing like little round doors. If your chakras *are* open and ready because you are physically, mentally, and spiritually balanced and strong, then you are ready for the transformative energy of *Kundalini*.

In Betsy's practice, she has not encountered anyone experiencing the rise of Kundalini. She believes this is because people typically come to her when they feel out of balance, physically and/or emotionally. We've already said this, but we want to emphasize it again: When we are in a state of imbalance, *Kundalini cannot rise*. Betsy also believes that the rising of this intense energy is a fairly rare occurrence. It is hard work to bring awareness and attention to one's own issues, and even harder to change those aspects of our lives that are not working. We all have "stuff"—baggage and issues that limit our potential. When we work through one layer of our "stuff," we often discover another layer, and another and another! This is normal, and it is part of our contract as human beings, to work through our issues so that we can be open vessels through which Kundalini energy can flow. But this may take a lifetime (or many lifetimes) of work! So stop worrying about Kundalini and start working on paving the way for her future passage.

Preparing the Body for *Kundalini*

One of the ways the practitioner of yoga prepares for spiritual awakening is by practicing the Eight Limbs of Yoga, also called *Ashtanga yoga*. (*Ashtanga* means eight limbs or eight parts.) Most yoga paths mention and recommend following the eight limbs, even though many Western yoga paths mostly emphasize just the third limb—the *asanas* or physical poses. These are important, but not the only aspect of yoga.

The purpose of the eight limbs, which we explained in Chapter 2, is to help the individual fully integrate with universal divinity. They are like stepping-stones to make it easier. There have been those few who manage to achieve enlightenment without necessarily following all these steps, but the point of the eight limbs is to prime the body, mind, and spirit. Think of it as taking singing lessons so you can sing better. Some people have amazing voices without lessons, but most of us can benefit from some instruction and a lot of practice.

The Eight Limbs of Yoga are all things you can do in your daily life. They comprise a whole-self workout plan, covering the behavior, the body, the breath, the mind, and the spirit. You can look back to Chapter 2 for more detail, but just as a quick review, the eight limbs are the *yamas* (healthy behaviors to practice, like nonviolence, truthfulness, and not stealing), the *niyamas* (things to observe, like cleanliness, inner contentment, and self-discipline), the *asanas* (the yoga poses), *pranayama* (breathing exercises), *pratyahara* (sensory withdrawal), *dharana* (concentration), *dhyana* (meditation), and *samadhi* (union with divine energy).

These are all goals to work toward, but this is good physical, mental, and spiritual work. The peripheral benefits of practicing the Eight Limbs of Yoga are amazing. You get physically and mentally stronger, calmer, more content, and more centered. The healthy open state of your chakras proves it. Regular practice of the eight limbs also primes your body, mind, and spirit for *Kundalini* to wake up and get moving.

But even then, *Kundalini* isn't going to just suddenly zip up your spine and turn you into some levitating guru right in the middle of your dinner meeting. You have to be working on it, and if you are working on it, you will be ready for it. (And even when it happens, we're sorry to say that you probably will not levitate.)

To get *Kundalini* to rise, then, is a long process of preparation. You might hear stories about people who experienced spontaneous *Kundalini* rising, but we believe that when this happens, it isn't as spontaneous as it might seem. Those people really were ready. Or, it wasn't *Kundalini* rising at all. It was something else. Rest assured that a focus on a healthy body and mind, which are reflected in strong, balanced, open chakras, is a safe, sound, and ultimately rewarding path.

How *Kundalini* Moves

When you get to that strong, balanced, healthy point (maybe you are already there), and you are practicing yoga or exercising regularly, eating a pure healthy diet, and spending time each day meditating or praying, *Kundalini* might begin to stir. It might happen during a yoga practice or especially if you are meditating.

When *Kundalini* begins to move, it feels like different things to different people. Some people experience a feeling of movement at the base of the spine, like a creeping or jumping feeling. Some feel heat in the spine. Others experience a flutter, or the sensation of cold in the lower back. Sometimes the feeling is dramatic, like your mind suddenly popping open. Sometimes the feeling is subtle, as if *Kundalini* has moved just a little. You might feel a rising sensation at the base of the spine that moves up the spine, or you might not feel much movement at all. The way Kundalini manifests for you depends on who you are, the state of your body and mind, and what you are prepared to experience.

Spinning Your Wheels

Betsy has a friend who began to notice snakes everywhere in her environment—not only real snakes, but also pictures, cartoons, TV commercials, and books about snakes. She was in the midst of deep spiritual work, and took these signs as proof that Kundalini was rising.

Whether the sensation is dramatic or not doesn't really matter. If you get too attached to the idea of making *Kundalini* move, you can throw yourself out of balance again. Remember, it is just you, waking up. When that happens, you will enjoy a creative surge like you've never experienced before. You might feel suddenly filled with love, or you might feel deeply connected to everyone around you. The feeling might last for a while, or it might be fleeting. Let yourself feel it and see where it takes you.

When *Kundalini* moves, it can feel exciting, or serene, or just interesting, but it's not going to change your personality. What it can do is show you the best aspects of your personality that you might not have been allowing full expression. Just remember, *Kundalini* is part of you. Work on yourself, and allow your best self to emerge. That's what it's really all about.

> ## !!! Wake-Up Call
>
> No matter how often we tell people not to worry about *Kundalini*, some people still do. They worry about feeling something foreign or scary or going to a mental or spiritual place they can't handle. The human mind is highly suggestible, but an authentic *Kundalini* experience is a beautiful thing. Personally, we believe that bad *Kundalini* experiences aren't *Kundalini* experiences, but not everybody agrees with us on this point. In any case, if you ever experience disturbing physical sensations, thoughts, or feelings that are violent, self-destructive, or frightening to you, don't try to deal with them alone. There are many wonderful, experienced therapists and health practitioners out there who can help you sort out what's going on.

Kundalini Transformation

People often wonder what happens to them *after Kundalini* wakes up. Will they be the same? Will they be normal? Or will they become all weird and nobody will be able to relate to them anymore? Fear not. Those who engage in serious spiritual work and finally do experience *Kundalini* awakening report surges of creativity, brilliance, engagement in the world, an ability to help others, and other wonderful results. Some people believe that *Kundalini* awakenings are the source of great artistic ability and genius. Many also believe that as more people experience *Kundalini* awakening, the human race will take an evolutionary leap forward.

Perhaps *Kundalini* is a catalyst for activating our higher selves. We see the world changing around us every day, in amazing and transformative ways. As Gandhi said, "Be the change you wish to see in the world." As you awaken through the help of your own *Kundalini* energy, you will have the energy, the vision, and the inspiration to be that change.

Getting Started with *Kundalini*

In addition to practicing the Eight Limbs of Yoga, there are some specific exercises you can do that tone your chakras and manipulate your *prana* in a way that can encourage *Kundalini* to awaken. You can do this in many ways, including the following two exercises.

Cobra Pose (*Bhujangasana*)

Yoga's Cobra pose evokes serpent power.

This simple yoga pose actually imitates the shape and movement of a snake—an apt pose for awakening the serpent power. Because *Kundalini* starts in your first chakra, this pose is effective because it concentrates energy in that first chakra. Here's how to do it:

1. Lie on a yoga mat or a folded blanket, on your stomach. Place your hands on either side of you, palms on the floor, at the level of your chest. Keep your elbows hugging into the sides of your body. Stretch your legs out behind you, and click your toenails into the mat.

2. Visualize your first chakra at the base of your spine. Press this area into the floor, along with the tops of your thighs, your knees, and the tops of your feet, so that your entire lower body feels rooted to the ground. Keep your tailbone tucked in to prevent low back pain. Everything from the hips down should be pressing into the floor, but especially feel the area around the first chakra, at the base of your tailbone, rooting down into the ground.

3. Inhale and begin to lift your chest off the floor. Gradually rise up, using your arms for support, until your arms are straight, or as straight as you can make them without putting any pressure on your back. Your lower back moves in and up.

4. Press your hands firmly into the mat, and imagine your hands moving back toward your hips as your heart and chest extend forward. Breathe normally and hold this position for 10 to 30 seconds, or as long as feels comfortable and energizing.

5. Exhale and slowly lower your chest and head back to the floor. Rest your forehead on the floor and breathe. Feel the energy accumulating in your first chakra. Repeat one or two more times.

Mula Bandha

Bandhas are locks inside the body that seal off the *nadis* to concentrate *prana*. The three primary locks used in yoga practice and Kundalini work are *mula bandha*, *uddiyana bandha*, and *jalandhara bandha*. This is key for energizing the chakras and awakening *Kundalini*. To understand how this works, it helps to understand that within the body, there are different kinds of *prana*.

Without getting too technical, a kind of sub-*prana* moves upward through the *sushumna nadi* when you inhale, and another type of *prana*, called *apana*, moves downward through the *sushumna nadi* when you exhale. When *prana* and *apana* meet, they create a spark, which can awaken *Kundalini*. Getting them to meet means infusing the body with *prana* and holding it inside.

def•i•ni•tion

Bandha is the Sanskrit word for lock, and *bandhas* are muscular contractions of the body practiced to hold energy or *prana* inside the body temporarily. There are three primary *bandhas*: **mula bandha,** or Root lock, a lock at the first chakra; **uddiyana bandha,** or Abdominal lock, a lock at the third chakra; and **jalandhara bandha,** or Throat lock, a lock at the fifth chakra.

Apana is a type of sub-*prana* that moves downward through *sushumna nadi* with exhalation. One of its functions is to move spent energy out of the body.

Mula bandha, or Root lock, is one of three primary *bandhas*. This one involves a muscular contraction of the pelvic floor, at the first chakra. Normally, *apana* moves downward, but with the first chakra locked, it gets trapped and moves back up, where it meets and mingles with *prana*. This causes a sort of combustion, an inner spark that can help to nudge *Kundalini* awake.

Regular practice of *mula bandha* can help your awareness expand beyond the boundaries of the physical world and material concerns, to a higher awareness. It's a powerful exercise, but it's not hard to do. Here's how to do it.

1. Sit comfortably on the floor on a folded blanket with your legs crossed and your spine straight. Breathe normally.

2. Focus your attention on the first chakra, at the base of your spine. Feel the muscles on your pelvic floor, all around the area where your body touches the blanket. Try to contract these muscles, as if pulling the first chakra inward and upward. Relax. Do this a few times, to get the feel of it. We don't want to offend anybody, but for the sake of being clear, this contraction is what you would do if you were urinating and wanted to stop the flow, at the same time contracting the muscles around your anus. (If you've ever been instructed on how to do Kegel exercises, do that. It's the same idea.) The movement is actually to contract and raise the entire pelvic floor, so your internal energy moves up instead of down.

3. Now, take a long, slow, gentle breath in. When you have filled up your lungs, hold your breath and engage those first-chakra muscles. Hold your breath for 5 to 10 seconds, then gently exhale. Release the lock. Repeat. Do this a few times every day, for maximum effect.

The Least You Need to Know

♦ *Kundalini* is the Sanskrit word for "coiled." It refers to the inner spiritual energy lying dormant in our first chakras. With proper preparation and techniques, we can awaken our *Kundalini* energy for greater creative ability and expanded spiritual awareness.

♦ *Kundalini* has a reputation for being dangerous, but with the right preparation, you have nothing to fear. *Kundalini* will only rise up through the body when you and your chakras are open, healthy, and ready for a spiritual experience.

♦ Regular practice of the Eight Limbs of Yoga primes the body, mind, and spirit for awakening *Kundalini*.

♦ Certain exercises like the Cobra pose and *mula bandha* can help to increase internal energy in a way that encourages *Kundalini* to awaken.

Chapter 6

Be Mindful of Your Chakras

In This Chapter

♦ Defining mindfulness

♦ Using mindfulness techniques to tune in to your chakras right now

♦ Scanning your mind-body for a chakra quick-check

♦ Measuring your chakras

"I think, therefore I am," wrote Descartes, the seventeenth-century French philosopher. Most of us have been raised to believe that we are our thoughts, for how can we ever separate ourselves from them? And yet, according to yoga philosophy, we are not our thoughts. Thoughts are something we have, like hands or hair or clothing, but they are not us. They are not *you*, or at least, they do not define you. They are not the *whole* you.

But it probably will be difficult for you to recognize the truth of this unless you practice *mindfulness*. Mindfulness is the act of paying attention without engaging in what you are paying attention to. In other words, mindfulness is awareness, pure and simple. It is not thought, but it is aware of thought. It is not feelings, but it is aware of feelings. It is not your physical body, but it is aware of your physical body. It is the ability to perceive yourself and all your qualities without making the mistake that you *are* any of your qualities. It is the you that transcends qualities. *Mindfulness meditation* is a specific technique to cultivate mindfulness, but you can be mindful anytime, anywhere. You just have to stop your chattering brain, take a deep breath, and *be*.

The Benefits of Mindfulness

Mindfulness isn't just helpful for meditation. It has tangible physical benefits. In fact, many doctors, psychologists, and health-care facilities teach and employ mindfulness techniques because of their proven stress-reducing effects. Mindfulness techniques, including mindfulness meditation, can significantly reduce blood pressure as well as muscle tension and stressful feelings, including anxiety.

Mindfulness can also improve your performance in all aspects of your life. If you are exercising, including doing yoga, mindfulness can reduce the risk of injury because you will be so keenly aware of your body and how it feels as you move it. In your work, mindfulness can aid in concentration, improving efficiency and quality of what you are doing. Your mind won't be wandering off to what you will do next or what you did before. Instead, you can experience total absorption in your task through mindfulness.

Why do we bring up mindfulness in this book? Because mindfulness is a key element in reading your own chakras. It's easy to imagine what your chakras might be doing, but through mindfulness, you can gain a more clear, unadorned perception of your chakras. Through mindfulness techniques, you can learn to feel your chakras, assess their current qualities, and even fix them.

(!!!) Wake-Up Call _____

> If you ever eat while watching television, or watch television while surfing the Internet, or surf the Internet while talking to your kids, you know about multitasking, but you may not know much about mindfulness. Beginning to eat a bag of chips and then suddenly realizing the entire bag of chips is gone is eating *without* mindfulness. When someone is talking to you and you suddenly realize your mind has been wandering (or focusing on your Facebook messages) and you didn't hear anything that person said to you, that is listening *without* mindfulness. In fact, multitasking is anti-mindfulness, so give yourself a break from it once in a while. When you need to do something, eat something, or listen to something, do that, and nothing else. Try it. You'll instantly get better at whatever you are doing.

Pay No Mind

Mindfulness takes some practice because most of us aren't used to paying attention to the present moment without letting our brains simultaneously wander elsewhere. Daily mindfulness practice helps to train your mind into increased awareness, and what better way to practice than by meeting and greeting your own chakras?

You don't have to get all meditative about mindfulness. In fact, you can have mindfulness moments throughout the day, whenever you choose to have them. Just stop what you are doing, disengage from your thoughts, and expand your awareness so that you look *at* your thoughts, feelings, and sensory perceptions without letting them rule you.

You can tune in to your chakras in this way throughout the day, too, especially if you notice a physical sensation in the area of a particular chakra. Got a sore throat, butterflies in your stomach, chest pain, an ache in your lower back? Bring your awareness to that area and without judgment, see if you can notice anything going on in your chakra.

But wait—tuning in to your chakras is pretty challenging work if you aren't even used to tuning in to your physical body. Chakras are part of your *energy body*, so they require even more finely honed perceptive powers.

def•i•ni•tion

Your **energy body** is part of you, but not part of your physical body. It is the layer of you consisting of the energy that flows in and around your body, through your *nadis*, and concentrates in your chakras.

Mindful Matters

This mindfulness exercise can be challenging, but we're confident you can give it a try. You may have a hard time the first time, but every time you practice this exercise, it will get easier. It's like a workout for your brain, and you get in better shape the more you practice.

1. Sit comfortably on a folded blanket, or even in a chair, as long as you are sitting upright and your spine is straight.

2. Lower your eyes to approximately a 45-degree angle, and soften your gaze so you aren't looking at anything. Closing your eyes makes it easier for your mind to wander.

3. Withdraw your awareness from your thoughts. In other words, step back mentally from your thoughts and look at them, as if they belonged to someone else. Don't expect them to stop, because they won't. Just look at them. For example, you might notice that you are thinking about whether you can do this exercise or not. That's a thought. Visualize wrapping it up inside a bubble and labeling it: *thought.*

4. Now, expand your awareness to your physical body. Notice how it feels, as if someone else were telling you about it, as in, "That person's knee itches," or "That person's shoulders are rolling forward," or "That person is hungry." You can scratch your itches or adjust your posture if you want to (hold off on getting up to get something to eat for the moment!), but notice how it feels to do those things. Every physical sensation that you notice, visualize wrapping it up in a bubble and labeling it: *itch* or *shoulder roll* or *hunger.*

5. Now, expand your awareness to the room around you. What do you hear? How does the air feel on your skin, and how does the blanket feel underneath you? Do you smell anything? Notice what your senses perceive, but again, notice them as if they belonged to someone else. For every sensation, visualize wrapping it up in a bubble and labeling it: *cold* or *soft* or *radiator noise* or *burnt toast.*

6. Now, expand your awareness to your awareness. Has it shrunk down to the size of a thought? Step back again, out of your thoughts and your sensory perceptions. Mentally look at them all, as if they belonged to someone else. Now, try looking away from them. What is left to perceive, that is not thought or sensory perception?

7. Stay there as long as you can. When you get caught up in a thought or a feeling and it sweeps you away, notice it happening, and then step back off the ride, wrap it in a bubble, and label it. Then turn back around and step back into your unbridled awareness.

8. Try to stick with this for about five minutes. Repeat once or twice a day, and see if you can work up to 20 minutes.

Energy Unplugged

Your chakras tend to be open and strong after a yoga class, a massage, or energy work. When you are feeling particularly anxious or stressed, or just experienced something traumatic, your chakras tend to close temporarily. Chakras can change from day to day and moment to moment. Long-term patterns are more significant than a chakra's condition at any given moment.

Hello, Chakras!

After you have the concept of mindfulness in your head, you don't have to master it to start checking out your own chakras. Go ahead and try this exercise, even if the previous exercise was challenging.

We go into more detail about actually visualizing your chakras in Chapter 19. For now, we just want you to focus on your perceptions. Let your mind be open and unengaged, and see what happens when you focus your awareness on your chakras. Mindfulness is a process, not a goal, and this chakra introduction exercise is all part of that process.

1. Lie on the floor on your back, on a yoga mat or a folded blanket. Tuck your shoulder blades under you so your chest feels broad and open. Stretch your legs out as far as you can, then relax them. Adjust your arms so they are about a foot from the sides of your body, and rest your hands with palms facing up.

2. Take a moment to step into mindfulness mode. Disengage from your thoughts. Don't try to banish them, just step back out of them and look at them. Look at your physical sensations. Look at your sensory perceptions. Let them be, disengage, and avoid any judgments you may feel toward yourself.

3. When you feel like you have stepped back from your thoughts and sensory perceptions, bring awareness to the base of your spine and into your first chakra. You know, theoretically, that this chakra should be round, red, and turning like a wheel, but rather than just imagining it, try to feel and perceive it with your awareness.

4. As you bring your awareness to your chakra, continue to let your thoughts come and go, as they will, but let your chakra be the focus of your concentration. Let images, feelings, and other sensory perceptions come to you. Don't judge what happens or try to control it. Remember, you are standing back and being mindful, not immersing yourself in thoughts or feelings right now. Just *notice*. You might get some images or feelings, or maybe you won't. Just let whatever happens, happen.

5. Now, shift your awareness to your second chakra. You know it should be round, orange, and turning like a wheel, but again, rather than imagining how it should look, try to feel and perceive what is really going on in there, just behind your navel. Mentally record your perceptions.

6. Move your awareness to each chakra, in order: to your yellow third chakra under your rib cage; to your green fourth chakra at your heart; to your blue fifth chakra in your throat; to your indigo/purple sixth chakra in your forehead; and to your purple or white seventh chakra at the crown of your head. Spend some time contemplating each one, without judgment. Just perceive.

7. After you've finished perceiving each chakra with awareness, slowly wiggle your fingers and toes, bringing your awareness back to your physical body. Roll to your right side, and when you are ready, sit up.

8. Write down your perceptions about your chakras right away, before you forget. If you've already forgotten, that's okay. The exercise is the important part right now. (However, next time, you can also get up and write down what you perceive after each chakra, instead of waiting until the end, if you really want a written record of the experience.) Record any sensory perceptions or thoughts you had about each chakra. Your perceptions are unique to you, so don't worry about what they are supposed to be. Just consider what they *are*.

9. Repeat this exercise at least once a week, so you can begin to perceive patterns in your chakras, such as which ones tend to be more noticeable to you, and which ones you have a hard time perceiving.

!!! **Wake-Up Call**

Some people find mindfulness exercises easy, but for others, they are incredibly challenging, especially when attempting to perceive subtle nonphysical phenomena like the chakras. If you try the chakra mindfulness exercise in this chapter and you don't feel or see or perceive anything, don't worry. Try again later. The more you get comfortable with the notion of mindfulness and of perceiving your own chakras, the easier the perceptions will come. Massage therapists and energy workers often have the ability to tune in to your energy and provide feedback about the health of your chakras. You might also consider enlisting a particularly intuitive friend, who might be able to meditate on and perceive qualities of your chakras for you. Later, as you hone your mindfulness skills, you can return the favor.

If you enjoy using mindfulness meditation techniques and want to establish a regular mindfulness practice, read more in *The Complete Idiot's Guide to Mindfulness* by Anne Ihnen, Ph.D., and Carolyn Flynn.

Measure for Measure

After you start tuning in to your own chakras, things start to get interesting. Suddenly, you have a tool for determining what aspects of your life are working well, and which ones need more attention (or less attention). Here's another tool for you: you can actually measure your own chakras.

When you measure your chakras, you can see exactly how big they are, what shape they are, and which direction they are spinning. Betsy frequently measures her clients' chakras, taking a baseline measurement at the beginning of therapy, then repeating the measurement on a periodic basis, such as weekly or monthly, to see what changes. Betsy explains that a single reading isn't necessarily significant. Chakras change from day to day, even from moment to moment. They can open and close, widen and narrow, change shape or position or direction of spin, then change back again, depending on what you are thinking, feeling, and experiencing at any given moment.

However, regular measuring can reveal more overarching patterns. For instance, a closed fourth chakra during a single measuring session doesn't necessarily mean that person is having issues with their heart. However, a persistently closed fourth chakra session after session is more telling. Perhaps that person has closed herself off from feeling love and compassion for others or refuses to care of herself.

To measure your chakras, you need just two things: a *pendulum* and a partner. You can buy pendulums, but you can also use a necklace with a weighty pendant on it. A tiny charm probably isn't heavy enough. The pendant should weigh more than the chain or cord on which it hangs.

Your partner should be a relatively disinterested person. In other words, he or she should not care what your chakras are like. If you have an emotional relationship with someone, especially if that person has strong opinions about which of your chakras will probably be open or closed, that person is not a good choice for this exercise. Choose someone who is open to the idea of measuring your chakras, but has no stake in the information.

def•i•ni•tion

A **pendulum** is an object hanging from a chain, cord, or other similar apparatus, that can swing freely. Pendulums can be used as tools for measuring the chakras because they swing freely and can therefore be influenced by the chakra's energy, in a way similar to the way a wind chime or mobile is affected by air currents.

Grounding Your Partner

Before you and your partner begin the chakra-measuring process, your partner must get grounded and separate her energy from yours. This is how Betsy suggests you can accomplish this:

1. You lie down on your back, on a bed or on the floor, on a yoga mat or a folded blanket. Ask your partner to stand or kneel beside you.

2. Your partner can now close her eyes and imagine her own energy rooting her down into the ground. She can visualize roots coming out of her feet or legs and anchoring her to the earth.

3. Next, your partner can open her eyes but visualize a heavy curtain of energy falling between the two of you. She can put her hand through it, but the rest of her body must stay on one side of the curtain, while your body stays on the other side. Mentally, your partner can say to herself, "I am detached from outcomes. What is hers is hers, what is mine is mine, and nothing crosses the curtain. My stuff stays on my side, and her stuff stays on her side." This separates your energy so the pendulum can read your energy and not your partner's energy.

Energy Unplugged

Some people wonder, if chakras pour out so much energy they can influence a pendulum, why would you need another person to hold the pendulum? It's true that if you were to hang a pendulum from an inanimate object over someone's chakra, it would not spin. The pendulum must be in contact with energy to conduct energy. A wire can't transfer electricity unless it is connected on both ends, and although *prana* is a little bit different than electrical energy (for example, the pendulum doesn't have to touch you to pick up your chakra energy pattern), the concept is similar. Your partner is the energizing force that powers the pendulum to be able to pick up your chakra's energy flow pattern.

How to Measure Your Chakras

When your partner is grounded, it's your turn to relax. Lie back and let the weight of the bed or floor support you. Breathe normally and close your eyes. Then, follow these steps to actually measure your chakras:

- With the pendulum in her dominant hand, your partner can now hold the pendulum by its cord about 2 feet above your body, which will be above your energy field. Your partner then moves the pendulum above your first chakra (at the base of your spine) and lowers it straight down to about 2 to 3 inches above your first chakra, which should bring the pendulum into the energy field of that chakra. Your partner should try to keep her hand as steady as possible and hold the pendulum with a loose grip rather than with a firm and rigid hold, which could prevent the pendulum from spinning in response to the chakra energy. Have your friend concentrate on keeping her own energy to herself, so she doesn't influence the pendulum. You want your own chakra energy to get it spinning, not hers.

♦ In most cases, the pendulum starts to swing. The shape of the swing and the direction indicate the shape and direction of your chakra's energy flow. You can both look at it, but try to stay still and centered. If the pendulum does not move, try moving it closer to your body. Or the chakra you are measuring may be closed. Remember, that might be just a momentary reaction. Sometimes people get nervous about having their chakras measured, and all the chakras clamp shut. Try to relax. This is supposed to be fun!

Measuring the Heart chakra.

♦ After you have determined the general state of your first chakra, your partner should lift the pendulum up about 2 feet, back out of the energy field, and with her other hand stop the swing. Now, she can bring it over the second chakra, around the navel area, and again, lower it straight down to about 2 to 3 inches over the chakra. Wait for the pendulum to start swinging.

♦ Repeat this process over each of the other chakras: the third chakra at the solar plexus, the fourth chakra at the heart, the fifth chakra at the throat, the sixth chakra at the forehead, and the seventh chakra about 2 inches above the crown of the head (so the pendulum will not actually be over your body, but rather 2 inches taller than the top of your head).

♦ Now it is your partner's turn. You try it on her.

What Do the Measurements Mean?

Now that you've watched the pendulum swinging in response to your energy fields and your friend's, you can interpret the results. Here are some guidelines to help you understand what your measurements mean:

- *Movement:* Once the pendulum is brought into the energy field of the chakra, the pendulum will start to move if the chakra is open. If there is no movement of the pendulum and it is about 1 to 2 inches above the body, this likely means that the chakra is blocked or closed.

- *Direction:* A healthy chakra should spin in a clockwise direction. If the pendulum is going back and forth, it may mean that the chakra is skewed in an oblong shape, which could mean the chakra is taking in energy sporadically. A right-left swing could mean that chakra is more skewed toward its physical aspects. An up-down swing could indicate that chakra is more skewed toward its psychological or spiritual aspects (see Chapters 7 through 13 for more on the physical and psychological/spiritual aspects of each chakra). If the pendulum goes counterclockwise, it could mean that chakra is closed, or that chakra is releasing energy instead of taking it in.

- *Diameter:* Ideally, all of your chakras are spinning in the same direction with the same diameter. This indicates balance. The diameter or distance across the circle created by the pendulum's spin should, in general, be about 4 to 6 inches. If it is less than this, it might mean the chakra is open but weak. If the diameter is greater than 6 inches, this usually signifies an excessive chakra that is overloaded with energy. You may find that if one of your chakras is excessive, the chakras on either side of it will measure a bit deficient or small.

Remember, a single measurement doesn't mean much. Measuring your chakras is best for establishing long-term patterns. However, a single measurement can be good at helping you to assess your mood or feelings at the moment. Maybe your second chakra is temporarily huge, and this helps you realize you are being overly emotional about something. Or maybe your first chakra is closed and this helps you recognize that you are feeling insecure or unsafe about something.

Mindful attention to your chakras is fun, interesting, and helpful in so many ways that we think it is well worth a few minutes out of your day. Tune in, and see where you are. You'll begin to achieve a whole new level of self-awareness.

The Least You Need to Know

◆ Mindfulness is the state of awareness, separate from (but noticing) thoughts, feelings, and sensory perceptions.

◆ Mindfulness techniques like meditation can help you tune in to the state of your own chakras.

◆ With a partner and a pendulum, you can measure your own chakras to assess their qualities at any given moment, including their size, direction and speed of spin, and alignment.

Part 3

Know Your Chakras: Bottoms Up!

This part is the heart of the book. We begin at the bottom with the first chakra and work our way up, chapter by chapter, through the chakras. From the Root chakra at the base of your spine, where your survival instincts and sense of security reside, all the way up to your Crown chakra at the crown of your head, where you connect with something greater than yourself, you learn what's going on inside each one, gaining a more intimate knowledge of your own physical and psychological issues. This part has the tools you need to awaken, align, energize, and even heal your chakras, one by one.

Root Chakra (*Muladhara*): Sleeping Power

In This Chapter

- ◆ What your Root chakra does, even without your help
- ◆ What your Root chakra represents for your body, mind, and spirit
- ◆ How to tune in to your Root chakra
- ◆ Correcting Root chakra blocks and overloads
- ◆ Using yoga for Root chakra fitness

They say every story has a beginning, a middle, and an end. For you and your story, your first chakra or Root chakra is your personal beginning. This is the place where you commence, as an individual, and this chakra begins to form while you are still in the womb, not long before birth. Here lies your sense of security, belonging, well-being, physical health, and prosperity. This is where you become grounded, and everything that happens in your body, your mind, and your spirit finds its source here.

The Root chakra (Muladhara).

Although the higher chakras are more spiritual, we would argue that in many ways, the Root chakra is the most important of all the chakras because without a strong, healthy Root chakra, it is difficult to maximize your potential in any area of your life. It is nearly impossible to achieve spiritual enlightenment without the steady, stable energy of your first chakra. A tree can't thrive, live, or even stay upright without roots, and that's exactly what your first chakra is for you: your roots. Without a strong and open first chakra, the first storm to come along would uproot us.

Root Chakra 101

Whether you notice it, work with it, or ignore it, your first chakra is always right there at the base of your spine, spinning its energy and trying to keep you grounded. Sometimes this chakra might grow larger with excessive energy and sometimes it might grow smaller or even close down for awhile, but it is consistently the root of your energy body, the sleeping spot for your *Kundalini* energy, and the measure of your sense of security, physical sensations, and place in the world.

The first chakra, also sometimes called the Root chakra or Earth chakra, is called *Muladhara* in the traditional Sanskrit, which means root or base support. It is associated with the Earth element because it represents the actual, physical connection to Earth and physical incarnation in a body. Its symbolic color is red and the traditional lotus symbol depicting this chakra has four petals. The sound associated with this chakra is the seed sound *LANG*. Chanting this sound helps to activate the first chakra.

This chakra is located at the base of your spine, in the area of your perineum. It is associated with several physical structures in the body: the coccygeal nerve plexus, the adrenal glands, the sacrum, and the organs that govern the elimination of waste from the body, particularly the anus.

Your Root chakra governs several very important aspects of your life, so let's look at them, one at a time.

The Three S's: Security, Safety, and Survival

We all come into this world in a vulnerable state, totally dependent on others for survival—and so begins our quest for security, a quest that will last a lifetime and originates in the Root chakra. Some people simply feel safe in the world and as if they belong, no matter what happens to them. Others always seem to have a gnawing sense of impending doom, and may even want to escape from life.

These feelings are reflected in the state of your Root chakra, revealing how secure you feel in your life, and even in your body. Are you safe? Do you have the basic requirements for survival, such as food and shelter? You probably do, and you may know this rationally, but you may not always trust or believe that you do, and that's a first chakra issue.

Energy Unplugged

First chakra security issues often stem from childhood experiences. If you didn't feel protected or were mistreated as a child, you probably have first chakra issues now. Birth trauma or a lack of good bonding with a mother figure in the early months of your life can wreak serious damage to a first chakra. If your parents didn't feel safe or secure while you were growing up, you may have inherited that internal sense of unease. On the other hand, if you felt safe and sheltered as a child and all your needs were met, from food and shelter to love and attention, you are more likely to have a strong and open first chakra as an adult.

Grounded for Life

Betsy encounters many clients in her practice with grounding issues, so this is something she often focuses on in treatment. Being grounded means feeling connected to the earth, comfortable in your body, and present in your physical surroundings—all signs of a healthy Root chakra. People who are grounded recognize that they live in a body and have to take care of their bodies, their homes, their cars, their bank accounts, and all the other aspects of life in the physical world. Being grounded gives you a firm foundation on which to build a life. The most spiritual person in the world won't get very far without also being grounded. The reality is that we may be spiritual beings, but we are in human bodies and we need to care for them.

Spinning Your Wheels _____

One of Betsy's clients, a young woman with an amazing talent for writing, was full of creative ideas but couldn't ever seem to manifest them. She lived in her own creative world in her head, but had difficulty managing finances, remembering to eat, or putting her brilliant ideas onto paper. During therapy, Betsy asked her client to take off her shoes, put her feet on the ground, and describe how the floor felt against the soles of her feet. Bare feet on the floor, the client admitted that she couldn't feel the floor at all. This was a sure sign that her first chakra needed work!

People who aren't grounded tend to be flighty, anxious, detached, and have little sense of their own bodies or how best to function in the physical world. Some of the most effective first-chakra healing exercises have to do with grounding. We talk about those later in this chapter.

Family Matters

An important part of each person's sense of belonging in the world is directly related to family, and also to what author and *medical intuitive* Caroline Myss refers to as tribe. Your family is your tribe (like it or not), but you may have other tribes as well, such as your friends, the people you work with, or other groups who share common interests or life experiences with you. Your country can be your tribe, generating feelings of patriotism. Your ethnic group, your gender, your neighborhood, or that tight-knit group of friends you've known since high school are all examples of different tribes you might claim as your own. When your tribe changes because of a move, a divorce, or a new job, you may encounter a period of first chakra upheaval until you settle into a new tribe and can establish new roots.

def•i•ni•tion

A **medical intuitive** is a person with the ability to use their own intuition to determine specific physical, emotional, or psychological illnesses or imbalances in another person. Sometimes, medical intuitives "see" a specific problem, such as a cancerous tumor in a particular place. Sometimes they simply get a sense of what the problem is, or even feel the same pain in their own bodies.

Your feelings about your place in your own family and your own tribe are reflected in your Root chakra, and can include feelings like patriotism and loyalty. Do you know that feeling you get when someone insults one of your family members or friends? That feeling of anger that says: nobody better say anything against my mother/father/brother/sister/friend/husband/wife/child, my dog/cat, or part of town/ethnic group/religion/country? That instinctual reaction comes from the first chakra.

Boundaries

The first chakra not only reflects your feelings of belonging in a group, but also sets boundaries that separate you from the other members of the group. You know where you end and others begin. First chakra problems are often related to boundary issues—people who are too open to others at their own expense, or are so closed to people that they never develop genuine and close relationships.

Prosperity Starts Here

How you handle your money, pay your bills, and save for the future are all aspects tied to your first chakra. People with strong first chakras tend to have a good grasp of what money represents (security and the ability to meet basic needs), and handle their finances in an organized and rational way. People with constant financial worries and irresponsible financial behavior often have blocked first chakras, whereas people who hoard money or are obsessed with material gain tend to have overloaded first chakras.

Energy Unplugged

Getting control of your financial life isn't quite as easy as opening up your first chakra. Keep making the same mistakes and your first chakra will keep closing up again. Instead, think about what ideas you have, perhaps inherited from your parents or related to impressions from childhood, that make you feel like you can't control your money, or that having enough money is somehow a bad thing. Examine these ideas, and what you *think* about money versus what you actually know to be *true* about money. Have your ideas about money been negatively impacting your financial life? Consider whether those ideas might be misconceptions.

Your Body, Your Health

The first chakra represents the physical aspect of you—your body. That means the condition of your body, your body image, your physical health, and your weight are directly tied to your Root chakra. When you are healthy and fit, you are in a better position to feel safe and secure, and to meet your own basic needs. When you are ill or unfit, you may feel less secure and less able to master your own survival needs.

Root Chakra Correspondences

Every one of your chakras corresponds not only to a particular color and sound but to a part of your body, a part of your mind, and a part of your emotional life. We'll go into more detail throughout this chapter about the many ways your first chakra speaks to you, but the following chart will lay it all out for you in a nutshell.

First Chakra	
Sanskrit name	*Muladhara* (root or base support)
Element	Earth
Color	Red
Seed sound	*LANG*
Location	At the base of the spine
Associated cultural phrases	"You have your two feet on the ground." "I'm putting my foot down." "Stand your ground!" "Take a stand." "I can't stand that." "What do you stand for? I understand."
Associated anatomy	Sacrum, coccygeal nerve plexus, adrenal glands, feet, legs, hips, bones, large intestine, anus, and skin.
Associated psychological and life issues	Security, safety, survival, being grounded, family and tribe (patriotism, loyalty), financial issues, health, body image, and weight.

Physical issues related to a blocked first chakra	Constantly getting sick, insomnia, endless dieting, anorexia nervosa, constipation, any disorders of the large intestine or problems related to the bowels, pain in the feet or legs, hip pain, any disorders of the bones, and skin problems such as lesions or breakouts.
Psychological issues related to a blocked first chakra	Fear, insecurity, flightiness, anxiety, inability to focus, disorganization, poor self-discipline, poor boundaries, poor sense of self, financial problems, and separation or dissociation from the body.
Physical issues related to an overloaded first chakra	Obesity, overeating, addictions, sleeping too much, fatigue, low energy, inability to move gracefully, plodding movements, and heavy feet.
Psychological issues related to an overloaded first chakra	Greed, materialism, obsession with money, inability to be generous, hoarding, workaholism, obsession with routines and security, fear of change, and overly strict boundaries/refusal to be open to others.
First chakra therapy	Eating protein and root vegetables, sleeping enough but not too much, massage, physical exercise, going barefoot, being outdoors, lying on the ground, and yoga poses that emphasize a firm base.

Awakening the Root Chakra

Before you open any of your other chakras, you must open this one, the place where your *Kundalini* energy lies sleeping. Awakening the Root chakra is easy to do. Vibration, movement, touch, exercise—anything physical awakens this grounded, centering chakra. Healing the first chakra will increase vitality and general energy, as well as help you feel more secure and less anxious.

To awaken your Root chakra, try this exercise:

1. Sit on the floor, legs crossed, seat firmly planted on the floor. Feel your pelvic bones and imagine roots anchoring those bones to the earth.

2. Take several long, slow, deep breaths as you visualize your deep red spinning first chakra, open and healthy at the base of your spine.

3. Imagine your chakra radiating a wide red beam of light from the base of your spine down into the floor, into the earth, and all the way to the center of the planet.

4. Imagine dropping an anchor from the center of your first chakra, slowly down into the center of the planet, and anchoring your body there.

5. Take a deep breath in and in a low resonating tone, say the word: *LANG*, holding the "A" sound (pronounced "ah," the word rhymes with "song"). Imagine the planet's energy beaming back up into your first chakra in a mutual exchange of energy that ignites your first chakra so that it glows gently as it spins.

6. As you imagine your first chakra heating up, continue to connect to the center of the earth and let yourself relax into a feeling of safety and security.

Aligning the Root Chakra

Crooked roots grow a crooked tree, so to make sure your Root chakra is properly aligned, try this exercise:

1. Stand in bare feet with your feet about hip-width apart. Feel the soles of your feet against the ground. Imagine your feet rooting firmly into the ground, as if magnetized to the floor.

2. Imagine your first chakra at the base of your spine and try to feel it spinning. Imagine a ray of light emanating down from your first chakra, through the floor. Then, imagine that same ray of light radiating upward, straight through the

crown of your head, pulling all your other chakras in line with this central column of light.

3. Lift your arms straight up overhead and imagine the red light pulsing up and down, reading to the center of the earth and all the way to the sky. Your chakra should now be aligned.

Blocks in the Root Chakra

As we mentioned earlier, Betsy encounters many clients with underactive or blocked first chakras. You may be able to spot this type of person on the street. They are the ones with darting eyes and uneven movements, and those who appear detached from this world. They are so in their heads that they may be the person walking across the street oblivious to the honking car racing toward them.

Childhood trauma or abuse is a common cause of first chakra blockage. Being neglected or lacking a strong bond with a parental figure early in life can also block a first chakra. If you didn't feel safe as you were growing up, it is difficult to feel safe as an adult, without some help. However, even if you weren't abused as a child, you may feel insecure in your first chakra, especially if you've had some financial problems, housing issues, health problems, or family problems.

Any one of these events can trigger the beginning of a series of events that can cascade into an energy imbalance, reflected in a first chakra that closes up defensively. When your first chakra stops the flow of energy, right at the root, you can experience a whole host of physical and psychological issues.

Blocked Chakra Health Issues

In particular, first chakra physical problems can be tied to the feet, legs, hips, and bones—the skeleton that supports you. Conditions that involve tightness are usually associated with the first chakra, like lower back problems, constipation, and difficulty having an orgasm. People who get sick all the time and generally have low energy often have first chakra blocks. So do people with eating disorders, excessive weight loss, and anxiety. Insomnia is generally caused by stress and tension, and those who suffer from it are prone to lying in bed caught in their head, thinking of everything that happened that day and everything that needs to be completed tomorrow. If an insomniac can work on becoming grounded into their first chakra while lying in bed, sweet sleep often follows.

Sometimes, your first chakra will close up temporarily in an unsecure situation, such as when you are traveling. This is why so many people experience constipation when they leave home. Their first chakras close tightly as if to say: *Nothing's coming out of this end. We're all sealed up and safe, thanks.* In these cases, be sure you are still taking care of your basic needs and spend some extra time getting exercise. Even if you aren't home, you can still focus on being in your body, with both feet on the ground.

> **Energy Unplugged** _____
>
> To alleviate temporary first chakra blocks while traveling, take a few minutes to meditate on how your body feels. Are you holding tension in your shoulders? Furrowing your brow? Is your neck stiff from a long plane ride? Lie on the floor for a few minutes and concentrate on relaxing anxious muscles and focusing on the feel of the earth beneath you. No matter where you are, you are always connected to the earth.

Blocked Chakra Psychological Issues

Psychologically, people with a blocked first chakra may be anxious, "wound tight," or may even feel a desire to detach completely from life. Detaching may mean avoiding friends, missing deadlines, or losing track of possessions; or it can be even more serious, where a person feels like they literally float away and leave their body. This type of detachment is often called dissociation, which is a disruption in a person's memory, identity, or perception of their environment, and usually warrants treatment by a professional.

Food addictions, alcoholism, and even workaholism are all complicated problems that involve multiple chakras; however, the first chakra is always a part of the equation. Addictions enable people to detach from a part of their life that is difficult or uncomfortable. Many people with an addiction admit that drinking or eating helps numb them and disconnect them from who they truly are.

Other issues related to first chakra blocks can include problems meeting your own basic needs, getting along with family members, and paying bills. It is very important for people with blocked first chakras to pay attention to basic self-care, such as personal hygiene, cleaning up the house, paying the bills, and taking care of the work of daily life in the world. First-chakra-blocked people have a hard time doing these things and may need to ask for help from a grounded friend to get organized. Getting into regular routines can make a big difference.

Healing a Blocked First Chakra

To heal and strengthen a blocked Root chakra, Betsy always encourages her clients to feel the floor. Take off your shoes and touch your feet to the ground. You can do this outside (weather permitting), but even bare feet on the floor of your home can be very grounding. Pay attention to how your feet feel against the floor. Walk on different surfaces and tune in to the varying sensations. Stand still and imagine roots growing down from your feet. Squat down if you feel steadier that way and imagine heavy weights in your feet, or magnets holding you to the surface of the earth.

Physical activity of any kind is also great for unblocking the first chakra. Anything that gets you out of your head and back into your body will help strengthen your foundation, such as …

♦ Eating, especially protein and root vegetables like potatoes, carrots, sweet potatoes, onions, and radishes; red foods like meat, beets, grapes, strawberries, and cherries also support a healthy first chakra.

♦ Sleeping more.

♦ Getting a massage.

♦ Taking a long, hot bath; washing your hair; washing your feet.

♦ Being outdoors in nature; connecting with the earth by walking in a forest, being barefoot on the beach; collecting pieces of nature to bring inside such as shells, leaves, and flowers.

♦ Exercising, including dancing, yoga, lifting weights, or just walking—anything that forces you to focus on being present in your own body.

♦ Consciously keeping both feet on the floor, preferably barefooted (if it's cold, put on some socks). Press both feet into the floor to strengthen your connection with the earth. Imagine you are trying to part the floorboards with your feet, or imagine the floor is made of sand and you are digging in.

♦ Using mantras to help train your mind and allow you to become more grounded into your first chakra. Mantras work best when repeated out loud prior to falling asleep and when first awakening. Examples of first chakra mantras: *My feet are firmly rooted to the earth. My body is well cared for and appreciated. The energy of the universe nurtures me. I feel at home in my body. My life is abundant. I am safe, strong, and alive.*

Energy Unplugged _____

An easy way to tune up your first chakra is to pay attention to your physical environment. What do you detect through your five senses? Stay quiet for a few minutes and note what you see, hear, smell, taste, and feel in your actual immediate surroundings—the right here, right now.

Overload in the Root Chakra

While first chakra blocks may be more common than first chakra overloads, the first chakra can certainly be prone to excess. First chakra overloads can be caused by too much routine, too little flexibility, too little change, boundaries that are too stiff, and a life void of spontaneity.

For some people, this pattern started in childhood. Maybe your upbringing was so rigid and rule-oriented that you aren't sure how to live any other way. Or maybe you had so few rules growing up that you over-reacted by imposing extremely rigid rules and boundaries for yourself in your daily life, and you are afraid to be too lax because that doesn't feel safe.

Overloaded Chakra Health Issues

The most common physical sign of an overloaded first chakra is obesity. Eating strengthens the first chakra, but some people go overboard and eat too much in order to feel heavier and more secure. For these people, losing weight isn't just a health issue; it feels like a threat to their own safety. They want to feel heavy and take up a lot of space, as a confirmation of their existence and place in the world. If you are very overweight, you may think you want to lose weight because, well … doesn't everyone? However, if you have an overloaded first chakra, you may not want to admit that being overweight really does feel safer to you.

Not all overloaded first chakra people are overweight, however. Some hyper-focus on their bodies to such an extent that they completely ignore other aspects of life, such as cultivating relationships or spirituality. These people tend to approach exercise and other physical pursuits in an extremely regimented fashion and can't go a day without exercising. They tend to have highly developed muscles and may be very physically healthy but are not balanced in other aspects of their lives.

Other more typical overloaded first chakra physical issues can include stiff ankles, knees, and hip joints, excessive fatigue, sluggishness, a heavy plodding gait, and the feeling that you just can't get moving.

> **(!!!)** **Wake-Up Call** _____
>
> If you are overweight, don't blame your first chakra. It reflects the imbalance that exists in your own energy field. To help repair your overloaded chakra, try moving more. Moving gets stagnant, pooled energy circulating through your body, which can make you feel better and set you on the right course for rebalancing your first chakra to be strong and healthy.

Overloaded Chakra Psychological Issues

Overloaded first chakras often result in people who hoard. They may overeat and become overweight, which is a form of hoarding food, but they may also hoard possessions and money, focusing so intensely on accumulating material wealth that they don't know how to give to others.

Overloaded first chakra people also tend to have a rigid sense of rules and boundaries, rarely allowing themselves to be vulnerable to other people or to act spontaneously. This extreme control keeps them feeling safe, but prevents them from experiencing genuine and open relationships, leading to loneliness and discontent.

A lack of spiritual beliefs or a sense of disconnection from anything "otherworldly" is often a hallmark of people with an overloaded first chakra. They tend to be so concrete that they have a hard time connecting with something larger.

Healing an Overloaded Root Chakra

Healing an overloaded Root chakra means draining some of that excessive physical energy, to make room for other kinds of energy, such as emotional and spiritual energy. Some of these strategies are the same as those needed to heal a blocked chakra, but the most important is to *move* the physical body because particularly earthbound people tend to have a hard time with movement and flexibility. Try activities such as …

- Exercises that increase heart rate, such as walking, running, or dancing.

- Jumping up and down, paying attention to the feel of hitting the earth and how that balances with the feel of freedom from the earth.

- Flowing styles of yoga such as *vinyasa*.

def•i•ni•tion _____

> **Vinyasa** is a Sanskrit word commonly used to describe a style of Hatha yoga that links sequences of poses together in a flowing motion, rather than holding poses for long periods.

◆ Stretching exercises, to increase range of motion in muscles and joints.

◆ Massage, including foot massage, which can get energy moving and flowing out.

◆ Eating lighter, airier foods such as leafy greens and fruit.

Yoga Poses to Balance the Root Chakra

The best yoga poses for balancing both blocked and overloaded Root chakras are those poses that help encourage your connection with the earth in addition to your flexibility above it. These poses encourage you not only to be rooted, but also to grow up and out from those roots into your full flowering.

Mountain Pose, or *Tadasana*

The Root chakra in Mountain pose (Tadasana).

Mountain pose is one of the simplest and most effective Root chakra-balancing poses. Just as the first chakra is the foundation of the body's energy system, *Tadasana*, or Mountain pose, is the foundation of all the other yoga standing poses, no matter how advanced. Here's how to do it:

1. Stand in bare feet with your feet hip-width apart. Inhale and feel your muscles soften as you open your mind and heart to Grace.

2. Place your feet parallel. Imagine a line running from the center of your ankle to your second toe on each foot, and make sure these two lines are parallel Lift and spread your toes and experience muscular energy in your legs. Feel all four corners of your feet touching the earth: the top outside corner, the outside heel, the top inside corner (the ball of your foot), and the inside heel. Press all parts of your feet into the floor evenly.

3. Inhale and move your upper inner thighs back and apart. Keeping this, scoop your tailbone down and forward while drawing your lower belly in and up toward your navel.

4. Imagine the crown of your head rising straight up to the sky and your spine lengthening, as the muscular energy in your legs powers down into the earth.

5. Breathe slowly and evenly as you imagine your feet sinking deeply into the earth, becoming part of the earth, so that you stand as firm and strong as a mountain.

Tree Pose, or *Vrksasana*

Tree pose is meant to represent a tree with roots deep in the earth and branches out-stretched in air, bringing perfect balance to the body and mind. To balance in this pose, of course, you need a solid and open first chakra. You may need to do this pose while holding on to the wall or a chair at first, but if you work on it regularly, you will probably eventually be able to balance on one foot in the full pose, without assistance. Practice hones the first chakra as well as the pose itself.

1. Stand in *Tadasana* (described above). Take a deep breath, and allow your mind and body to relax.

2. Shift your weight to your left foot and imagine your left foot sprouting roots that grow deep down into the floor below you. Concentrate on feeling all four corners of your foot against the floor. If your foot turns in, try lifting up the arch of your foot for a more stable foundation.

*Moving into Tree pose is a
rooting experience.*

3. Breathe in and lift your right foot up off the floor. Take hold of it with your right
   hand. If you have trouble standing on one foot (a common problem for people
   with blocked first chakras), you can hold on to a wall or a chair with your other
   hand to support yourself.

4. Put the sole of your right foot against the inside of your upper left thigh. If you
   can't quite reach your thigh, rest the sole of your foot against the inside of your
   left calf muscle. Don't rest your foot on your knee, which can put pressure on
   this sensitive joint. Note: this is easier if your legs and feet are bare. Fabric can
   make your leg too slippery. This pose is also easier if you angle your heel slightly
   forward, which might give your foot a better grip. If you can't keep your foot
   against your leg without help, you can hold your foot in place with your right
   hand.

5. To counteract the push of your right foot against your left leg, subtly shift your
   left hip toward the midline of your body so you are standing with hips level
   Firmly push your right foot into your upper left thigh, as your upper left thigh
   also pushes firmly into your right foot to provide stability.

6. Put your hands, palms together, in front of your heart. Breathe. If you can, slowly raise your hands up, separate your palms, and balance with both arms raised straight up overhead like the branches of a tree.

7. Lower slowly as you exhale. Repeat on the other side.

Corpse Pose, or *Savasana*

As you breathe out, feel your first chakra. Still, you are alive.

This pose, meant to imitate the utter stillness of a corpse, is traditional for rejuvenating the body after a rigorous yoga pose or practice, but you can practice it any time you need to get back in touch with the earth. This pose is excellent for grounding the first chakra because so much of your body literally touches the ground.

1. Lie on your back on the floor, or on a yoga mat. If it's more comfortable, you can place a folded blanket under your head, and/or cover yourself with a blanket.

2. Stretch both legs out as far as you can, then relax your legs completely.

3. Draw your shoulder blades onto your back, almost as if they are cradling your heart. Lift your chest, as your heart center shines out in gratitude for this opportunity to rest deeply. Rotate your arms so palms face the ceiling.

4. Adjust your head so it feels centered and comfortable.

5. Breathing slowly and in a relaxed, unforced away, close your eyes and concentrate on relaxing every part of your body, letting it melt down into the earth. Imagine the earth is holding you, supporting you, and keeping you safe. Let your brow, your temples, your jaw, even your scalp relax. Your eyelids feel heavy. Relax the muscles in your chest, stomach, arms, pelvis, and legs. Feel your entire back body sink into the yoga mat, making deep contact with the earth.

6. Imagine your first chakra glowing a deep red, slowly turning, and expanding as you let the earth's energy support you and flow into you. Hold the position for as long as you are comfortable, preferably for at least five minutes.

Partner *Savasana*

Enlist a partner or friend to help you experience even deeper levels of relaxation in *Savasana*. In this pose, a partner helps you move your thighs back to give you a deep sense of being grounded to the earth. When we are stressed, we unconsciously move our thighs forward. If our thighs can move into the back plane of the body, the entire body relaxes more deeply.

1. Set up in *Savasana* (as described previously).

2. Your partner stands above you with their feet straddling either side of your legs. With fingers spread and arms straight, your partner places their hands on your upper thighs, and begins to push your legs down more toward the mat. Your partner can put substantial weight and pressure on your upper thighs to help them move into the back plane.

3. If you want more grounding, you can have your partner "surf" on your upper thighs. The person in Savasana draws their arms into a 90 degree angle, with triceps pushing into the mat and palms facing up toward the ceiling. The partner places one foot on your upper thigh, close to where the leg meets the pelvis. The partner then places their hands on your hands, and steps the other foot up onto the other upper inner thigh. By continuing to hold your hands, the partner can balance or "surf" on your thighs. The additional weight of the partner on your upper thighs grounds them down, and you may experience a deep wave of relaxation. Hold the pose as long as you like, or as long as your partner can balance.

4. To get out of this pose, the partner continues holding your hands, and gently jumps both feet back to the floor at the same time.

Regular maintenance of your first chakra is incredibly important, not only for balance but to maintain your health and to keep you focused on the task of being in the body and taking care of life's work. You'll have plenty of time to focus on your other chakras and reap the benefits of balancing those, but until your first chakra is open, nothing else will work as well as possible. First chakra work is essential to the job of being human, so spend as much time working on this chakra as necessary. When *Kundalini* energy can flow cleanly and easily through your first chakra, you are on your way to the next stage of personal development.

The Least You Need to Know

♦ The condition of your first chakra represents your sense of security, safety, ability to survive, groundedness, your place in the family or tribe, financial state, and physical health.

♦ When the first chakra is blocked, symptoms include insecurity, fear, lack of personal boundaries, flightiness, anxiety, disorganization, financial problems, eating disorders, constipation, and problems with the feet, legs, hips, and bones.

♦ When the first chakra is overloaded, symptoms include hoarding, greed, materialism, obesity, overly strict boundaries, or obsession with the body.

♦ You can balance the first chakra by eating protein and root vegetables, sleeping more, getting massages, getting exercise, feeling your feet against the earth, and doing grounding yoga poses like Mountain pose, Tree pose, and Corpse pose.

Chapter 8

Passion Chakra (*Svadhisthana*): Go Create

In This Chapter

- ◆ What your Passion chakra does, even without your help
- ◆ What your Passion chakra represents for your body, mind, and spirit
- ◆ How to tune in to your Passion chakra
- ◆ Correcting Passion chakra deficiencies or excesses
- ◆ Using yoga for Passion chakra fitness

Everything you create, from a drawing or a poem to a strong emotion to an actual human being, is generated from energy that starts in your second chakra. The seat of your passions, this chakra governs your creativity, your sexuality, your fertility, and your most intimate relationships. This is where you *feel*. Indian artist and author Harish Johari writes that the second chakra moves "like a butterfly" and indeed, that feeling you get when you have "butterflies in your stomach" is your second chakra spinning with a particularly strong emotion.

When your Root chakra is strong, balanced, and open, your Passion chakra has the best chance at regulating your passions like a thermostat. Imbalances in the chakras directly below or above can sometimes force the second chakra to overcompensate, resulting in too much emotion ... or not enough. Always get grounded first, but once you have a firm foundation, you can do a lot with the powerful creative force of the second chakra.

Passion Chakra 101

The second chakra, also sometimes called the Passion, Sexuality, Sacral, or Water chakra, is called *Svadhisthana* in the traditional Sanskrit. This word is variously translated. Literally, it means "dwelling place of the self," but chakra expert Anodea Judith translates the word as "sweetness." The second chakra is associated with the water element because, in contrast to the first chakra's solid, grounded earthiness, the second chakra is filled with flowing, moving, watery energy, representing your connection with your own emotions and impulses to create. The second chakra's symbolic color is orange and the traditional lotus symbol depicting this chakra has six petals. The sound associated with this chakra is the seed sound *VANG*. Chanting this sound helps to activate the second chakra.

This chakra is located just below your belly button and radiates in and around your abdomen and your genitals, including the ovaries and uterus for women. This chakra is associated with several physical structures in the body in addition to genitals and organs of procreation, including the sacral nerve plexus, lower abdomen, lower back, appendix, bladder, kidneys, and hip area.

Your Passion chakra also has everything to do with some pretty interesting parts of you, so let's investigate.

Feeling It

Being able to feel emotions without becoming a slave to those emotions is an important part of psychological health, and that balance happens in the second chakra. In our culture, it's easy to believe you are your feelings, but feelings, emotions, and passions are just one part of the being that is you. Recognizing that feelings are something you *experience*, not something you *are*, is the key to emotional balance and a healthy, open second chakra.

The Passion chakra (Svadhisthana).

Of course, feelings and emotions are an important part of your whole self, but they are also seductive, and some people become addicted to the intensity strong emotions can bring. All emotions, such as jealousy, admiration, sexual attraction, revulsion, inspiration, or the feeling you get when you experience something pleasurable or painful, beautiful or disturbing, come from the second chakra. Learn to recognize them for what they are, and you are on your way to better balance.

Energy Unplugged

Children who don't get enough emotional attention from their parents, or who get too much from parents who are defined by or obsessively interested in their children, often have second chakra issues. So do children who were sexually or emotionally abused. Severe pleasure restrictions or not enough control over pleasures can also influence children as their second chakras are developing. Consider how your family handled emotions and love, to get an idea of your own second chakra issues. Was emotional expression suppressed or overexpressed in your home when you were growing up? If so, consider how you might be repeating these dysfunctional patterns in your adult life.

The One(s) You Love

The second chakra's passions extend most immediately to those we love the most. The fourth chakra (which we'll talk more about in Chapter 10) is the Heart chakra, sometimes called the love chakra; but our most intimate relationships start lower, at the second chakra. The feelings we get when we are physically, emotionally, and sexually attracted to someone happen here, and sometimes radiate through our entire bodies. Have you ever felt weak in the knees when you saw or even thought about the object of your desire? Your second chakra made that happen.

Of course, the natural culmination of sexual desire is sometimes reproduction, and that is a second chakra function, too. Our fertility is rooted in the second chakra, and by association, our deepest feelings for the children we produce come from the second chakra. Your fourth chakra helps you love yourself and the other beings on the planet, but your feelings for those special few that are almost a part of your own body are second chakra territory.

What About the Sex?

The second chakra is often called the Sexual chakra, and for good reason. Sexual desire starts here, and so do all the feelings of pleasure that come from that. Even when you are not involved in a meaningful emotional relationship, the second chakra still generates feelings of sexual attraction and pleasure, and that can be a problem for some people who get so addicted to that pleasure that they forget about the relationship part and just go for the sexual thrill. This is one sign of second chakra overload.

On the other hand, blocked second chakras can cause a different kind of sexual problem—*sexual arousal disorder*. Ideally, when the second chakra is open and healthy, sexual pleasure becomes one lovely part of an entire balanced set of passionate emotions.

def•i•ni•tion

Sexual arousal disorder is the inability to become aroused, sustain arousal, or experience orgasm during sexual activity. This can happen to men or women, and may have physical or psychological causes. In either case, this disorder is reflected in a blocked second chakra.

Fertility

Your second chakra reflects your fertility, and people with infertility problems typically have a blocked second chakra. Working to open the second chakra while in treatment for infertility can help to support your efforts to conceive. (See the sections later in this chapter for second-chakra-opening exercises.)

Spinning Your Wheels

Betsy has a female client with infertility, which is generally related to the second chakra where our reproductive organs are housed. She was the oldest daughter of a dysfunctional family, and she felt the responsibility of constantly picking up the pieces. Despite having several siblings, she was the one who planned and hosted the family dinners, took care of her ailing mom and dad, lent money to family members, and offered to take in a family member who had recently become homeless. She was constantly giving away her second chakra energy to her family of origin, and they were happy to take it. Because of this, she had little energy left in her second chakra to nurture the development of a new life to start her own family. Until she could develop better boundaries with her siblings and parents and learn how to say "no," Betsy explained that her beleaguered second chakra would remain weakened, which could be making conception more difficult.

Your Creative Spark

The second chakra gets a lot of press for being all about the sex, but another important part of your passionate self exists here, too—your creativity. Everything you create in your own mind comes out of this chakra. This is the chakra that generates your impulse to make art, write a poem, play music or sing, dance, design your own website or blog, decorate your living room, or get crafty with a scrapbook or a photo album.

A blocked second chakra can result in a creative block, but a healthy, open chakra often reflects an open, creative person who can become passionately absorbed in work, hobbies, or whatever other passions inspire the creative fire.

Energy Unplugged

Life gets busy, and making time for creativity can sometimes feel unnecessary. However, exercising your creative impulses is just as important as exercising your body and mind. You don't have to write the Great American Novel or paint a masterpiece to stay creatively charged. Something as simple as writing in a journal each night, doodling in a sketch book, or using computer software to design your dream house will make you a more open, flexible, and well-rounded human being.

Grace

You can spot a person with a healthy second chakra by the way she moves. Graceful, flowing, sensual bodies almost certainly contain strong, open second chakras. Consider how you move, and what that says about your second chakra. Clumsy, awkward, stiff, stilted movements are often a sign of a closed second chakra, while hyper-flexible limbs and a lot of back-and-forth movement while walking may be a sign that your second chakra is too open. Are you graceful or clumsy? Do you float or stomp? Purposefully moving in a more graceful way will, in turn, help to relax and open a closed second chakra.

Passion Chakra Correspondences

Your Passion chakra governs many aspects of your body as well as your mind and feelings. Check out the following chart for a summary of Passion chakra correspondences, then read on to find out more detail about the many ways in which your Passion chakra reflects and influences your life.

Second Chakra	
Sanskrit name	*Svadhisthana* (dwelling place of the self, sweetness)
Element	Water
Color	Orange
Seed sound	*VANG*
Location	Just below the belly-button, in the abdomen
Associated cultural phrases	"Listen to your gut." "I've got butterflies in my stomach!" "I have a funny feeling …."
Associated anatomy	Abdomen, sacral nerve plexus, genitals, reproductive organs, kidneys, bladder

Associated psychological and life issues	Passion, emotions, sexuality, creativity, intimate relationships, parenting issues
Physical issues related to second chakra blockage	Fertility problems, sexual arousal disorder, "nervous stomach," stiffness, stilted movements, bladder infections, kidney stones, skipped or stopped menstrual periods, lower back pain
Psychological issues related to second chakra blockage	Creative blocks, fear of relationships/commitment issues, emotional coldness, inability to experience pleasure, shallow relationships, communication problems with children
Physical issues related to second chakra overload	Emotional eating, sexual addiction, substance abuse, frequent urination, heavy menstrual flow, PMS, hyper-flexibility
Psychological issues related to second chakra overload	Bipolar disorder, panic attacks, excessive emotionality, mood swings, hypersensitivity, addiction to pleasure, emotional dependency, ruled by feelings, over-association (enmeshment) with children

continues

continued

Second Chakra	
Second chakra therapy	Drinking more fluids, swimming, treatment for addictions, balancing pleasure activities (increasing or decreasing), counseling for emotional, relationship, and/or sexual problems, moving and flowing exercises that increase grace, such as ballet and *Vinyasa* or other flow styles of yoga

Awakening the Passion Chakra

If your *Kundalini* energy is activated in your first chakra, then you can encourage it to rise up into your second chakra. When you awaken your Passion chakra, you are likely to experience more vivid and intense emotions, a higher level of creativity, and more intimate relationships. Your potential increases when this chakra is healthy. Awakening the Passion chakra is easy and pleasurable.

Anything that gets your body moving in a graceful, flowing way, or that puts you in direct contact with someone you love, can activate this chakra. Or combine the two: try dancing slowly in rhythm with your partner as you both look directly into each other's eyes. This exercise is intense for some people, but it should launch you right into second chakra arousal. Try it in a hot tub and … well, we can't be responsible for what might happen next!

To get more Passion chakra energy into your environment, highlight the color orange. Wear orange, paint your bedroom orange, or put orange flowers around the house. Just seeing the color can help to awaken this chakra. Also include more water elements in your home. Remember lava lamps? Those flowing water lights are not only groovy, they can encourage a more fluid mood. Fill up crystal bowls with water and float flower buds in them, or add a desktop fountain or aquarium to your home.

You can also try this exercise for awakening the Passion chakra:

1. Sit on the floor, legs crossed, seat firmly planted on the floor. Feel your pelvic bones and imagine roots anchoring those bones to the earth.

2. Take several long, slow, deep breaths, then draw your attention to the area just below your belly button. Imagine your second chakra, a bright fiery orange circle spinning slowly.

3. Imagine your chakra radiating an orange circle of watery light that encompasses your entire abdomen. Feel the warm light pulsing in waves like ripples in a pond that expand outward from your spine, flowing to the front of your body and all the way to the back of the body, as well as out to each side. Feel the warmth in your hips and genitals.

4. Take a deep breath in and in a low resonating tone, say the word: *VANG*, holding the "A" sound (pronounced "ah," the word rhymes with "song."). Imagine the orange light filling your entire body with slow, steady waves of warm water.

5. Continue to breathe and let the warm waves of emotion and pleasure continue to radiate from your second chakra, as long as you like, allowing yourself to bask in the warm pleasure of the second chakra.

Aligning the Passion Chakra

When waves hit the beach at a diagonal, the beach erodes. To make sure your Passion chakra is properly aligned, try this exercise:

1. Immerse yourself in warm water, either in a bathtub, hot tub, or even a natural body of water like a lake or the ocean on a warm day, if you are lucky enough to have access.

2. Sitting or standing in water at least up to your waist, imagine your second chakra just below your belly button, and try to feel it spinning. Imagine a ray of orange light emanating down into your first chakra, where it combines with the red light and beams down into the ground. Then, imagine that same ray of orange light radiating upward, straight through the crown of your head, pulling all your other chakras in line with this central column of light.

3. Lift your arms straight up overhead and imagine the orange light pulsing up and down, radiating to the center of the earth and all the way to the sky. Your chakra should now be aligned.

Blocks in the Passion Chakra

Although many people are in tune with their emotions, there are exceptions. If you grew up in an environment where emotional expression or pleasure seeking was discouraged, you may never have learned how to be emotionally open. Or if your upbringing was emotionally overwhelming—maybe one of your parents had emotional issues and subjected you to too much emotional energy—you may react by withdrawing your own emotions in order to protect yourself.

That in turn can block your ability to have intimate relationships. It can also block your creativity. People who think they "just aren't creative" are more likely to have blocked second chakras. Believe it or not, everybody is born with creative potential. It's just that we don't all get the chance to nurture this inborn quality.

Your second chakra can get blocked later in life, too. A particularly painful relationship or break-up can cause a temporary or long-term second chakra block, especially if you didn't get support for your feelings or were discouraged from expressing your feelings over the course of a relationship. Sexual rejection or sexual exploitation can cause serious second chakra issues. Naturally sensitive people are also more likely to experience pain associated with emotions, causing a chain reaction of emotional imbalance that can influence future relationships as well as the ability to experience pleasure.

Blocked Chakra Health Issues

Second chakra issues are largely centered around the sexual and reproductive organs. Infertility, skipped menstrual periods, and sexual arousal disorder can all be related to second chakra blocks. So can a so-called "nervous stomach," stiffness, stilted movements, bladder infections, kidney stones, and lower back pain.

Blocked Chakra Psychological Issues

Emotional blockages are at the heart of a blocked second chakra. Creative blocks, such as writer's block, are also common when this chakra is blocked. You may have a fear of relationships, commitment issues, and resistance to change. People might see you as emotionally cold, or you may only be able to maintain shallow relationships with other people, without true intimacy. You might also feel like you are unable or unworthy of experiencing pleasure. As a parent, a sign of a second chakra blockage is sometimes an inability or unwillingness to communicate with or bond with your children. However, this can also be a sign of second chakra overload, when your over-emotional attachment to your children makes *them* withdraw, creating the communication problem.

Energy Unplugged

Sometimes a painful emotional experience, such as the loss of a loved one, a break-up, or a big disappointment related to your creativity, can create a temporary second chakra blockage. This is the time to pay extra special attention to your own emotional needs. There is nothing wrong with allowing yourself a little extra pampering and pleasure, to help yourself heal and your second chakra to open again. Take long baths, have some ice cream, stay in and go to bed early. If you give yourself permission to grieve, but also permission to feel pleasure in your own way at your own pace, you can help your own second chakra to open up again.

Healing a Blocked Second Chakra

To heal and strengthen a blocked Passion chakra, Betsy encourages her clients to get in touch with their emotions. This can be a difficult task if it isn't something you typically do. Talking about your feelings with a close friend, confidant, or family member is a good way to release and express yourself. However, people with a blocked second chakra often don't have close relationships because they may have excessively high boundaries and difficulty connecting with others. Working with a trained counselor, therapist, or psychologist may be key to learning the skills of expressing emotions and connecting with others in a healthy and enjoyable way.

Moving in a graceful, flowing way is also great for unblocking the second chakra. Work with a movement therapist, or take a private yoga session with a teacher skilled in the connection between mind and body, to bring great healing to this chakra. Anything that gets your energies moving through and out of your body will help strengthen and validate your emotional and creative self, such as …

- Drinking lots of fluids, especially clean pure water.
- Eating orange foods like sweet potatoes, citrus fruits, salmon, papaya, and melon.
- Purposefully doing pleasurable things.
- Swimming, especially in clean natural bodies of water.
- Hugging someone who is emotionally open and cares about you.
- Talking about your feelings with a good listener.

- Creating something: drawing, writing, playing music, building, cooking.

- Spending time with your children and focusing on them, rather than being distracted while you are with them.

- Looking at someone who loves you directly in the eyes.

- Having sex with a caring and committed partner who is sensitive and responsive to your feelings.

- Exercising gracefully, including dancing (such as ballet) and flowing yoga (such as *Vinyasa* style).

- Movement-based therapy.

- Counseling for emotional, relationship, or sexual problems.

- Therapy for addictions.

- Reciting these mantras: *I am a desirable person. My feelings are good. It is safe to feel things. I create newness in my life. I feel pleasure in my relationships. I move easily and gracefully through life.*

Energy Unplugged

An easy way to tune up your second chakra is to pay attention to how other people feel. Sometimes what we see in others is a mirror for ourselves (psychologists call this projection), so tune in to people in your immediate environment. What do you notice about how others appear to feel? Especially notice the things that create an emotional response in you, whether it is sympathy or annoyance. Could that be a clue to how *you* are actually feeling?

Overload in the Passion Chakra

Why are you *so emotional?* Sometimes life demands an emotional response, but an overloaded second chakra can cause a host of problems, from mood swings and a general overly emotional reaction to things, all the way to full-blown addictions, codependency, or bipolar disorder.

Second chakra overload can happen when a naturally emotional person is encouraged to be that way early in life, by overly emotional or overly unemotional parents. Sometimes second chakra overload is a temporary response to an emotional situation, or simply a poor sense of how to regulate the eternal quest for pleasure. The result is emotion, emotion, emotion, and while overloaded second chakra people may be extra creative, they may also be so controlled by their feelings and passions that they completely lose their common sense.

Overloaded Chakra Health Issues

The most common physical signs of an overloaded second chakra are problems related to the sexual and reproductive organs. Heavy menstrual flow and severe PMS symptoms are signs of flooded second chakras. So is a high frequency of sexual arousal, especially coupled with the inability to control sexual conduct. Addictive behavior can be a sign of a second chakra flood, whether the addiction is to sex, food, alcohol, or caffeine.

Although eating is a classic first-chakra activity, overloaded second chakra people are prone to emotional eating and often become overweight because of this problem. Bulimia can be reflected in the second chakra, as people eat to dull strong emotions, then feel such strong guilt that they purge by vomiting or laxative abuse. Compulsive eating may be a first chakra problem, as people try to get heavier to get grounded, or a second chakra problem, when the eating is being used for the purpose of squelching strong feelings.

Other signs of an overloaded second chakra include severe PMS (especially mood swings, irritability, bloating, and abdominal cramps), and hypermobility and/or a wobbly or swaying walk. People with hyper-mobile joints and uncontrolled body movements are more prone to joint injury and osteoarthritis. This is often reflected in an overly open second chakra.

(!!!) Wake-Up Call

Got PMS? Try reining in your second chakra with more structure. Go to bed and get up on a regular schedule; eat regular, balanced meals;, and focus on deep breathing and temporarily removing yourself from a situation when emotions feel out of control. Drink plenty of water to battle bloating, and avoid mood enhancers like caffeine and alcohol, especially during that week before your period when you tend to have the worst symptoms.

Overloaded Chakra Psychological Issues

Overloaded second chakras can result in all kinds of destructive behaviors. This passion and pleasure center is easy to obsess about, and addiction to pleasure is a common problem. Sure, it might be fun to call yourself a hedonist, but if you can't stop a pleasurable behavior or if you gear your entire life around seeking pleasure, you are out of balance.

According to yoga philosophy, one of the primary reasons why people are hindered in their spiritual progress is through excessive attachment to pleasure, but even if spiritual progress isn't your goal, too much short-term pleasure seeking can seriously hinder your progress toward long-term goals. This can also lead to addiction, not to mention the destruction of relationships, the loss of your job, even the loss of your health.

The other way in which addictive behaviors are linked to overloaded second chakras is that people sometimes engage in these behaviors to mask uncomfortably strong emotions. If you are flooded with feelings and you don't know how to handle them, pleasurable behaviors can help dull the emotional pain. If you can't stop eating, smoking, drinking alcohol, taking recreational drugs, or seeking sex, you probably have a serious overloaded second chakra problem.

Issues of addiction typically require professional intervention. A medical doctor, therapist, or counselor can help you get back into balance if you can't stop doing something. There are too many good things in life to waste it all on an overloaded second chakra, so please get help if you can't help yourself.

Overloaded second chakra people also tend to be emotionally clingy, smothering the people they love and often losing them in the process. Balancing your second chakra can help you get a handle on the way you relate to other people, helping you to back off, balance your emotions, and listen a little more closely to your inner logical voice.

You have emotions so you can deepen your relationships, appreciate the good in the world, learn about yourself, be appropriately repulsed by the bad, and exercise your creativity, but you should be able to manage your emotions. They shouldn't manage you. Remember, you are not your feelings. You can set them aside, even discipline them, when they get in your way.

Healing an Overloaded Passion Chakra

Healing an overloaded Passion chakra means draining out some of that excessive passionate, emotional, creative energy, to make room for other kinds of energy, like grounding energy and spiritual energy. Creative, passionate energy is a good thing, of course—but it isn't the only kind of energy you need, so balance is best. Try strategies such as …

- Crafting a routine and sticking to it every day, especially in terms of when you sleep, eat, and bathe.

- Setting limits for yourself, especially regarding those things you like to do a little too much. If this is too difficult, enlist an accountability partner like a friend, co-worker, or therapist, who checks in with your progress

- Aerobic exercising, to burn off extra energy and help you feel pleasure in a healthy way.

- Strength training (lifting weights), to give support to a hyper-flexible body.

- Trying hot yoga styles, such as *Bikram* and Barkan, which are great for flushing excess water and emotions out of your body.

- Spending quiet time alone to focus on your own strengths and personal power, so you can feel more independent.

- Grounding exercises for the Root (first) chakra, and strengthening exercises for the Power (third) chakra.

def•i•ni•tion

Bikram yoga and other "hot yoga" styles are practiced in a room typically heated to around 100 degrees, with high humidity, similar to the climate in India, where yoga originated. This type of yoga induces sweating to purge toxins from the body. The heat also increases flexibility.

Yoga Poses to Balance the Passion Chakra

The best yoga poses for balancing both blocked and overloaded Passion chakras are those poses that help encourage graceful, flowing movements along with flexibility and strength. The classic moving sequence of poses for warming the body and increasing flexibility is called Sun Salutation, or *Surya Namaskar*.

Different teachers approach the sequence in different ways. Here is one flowing sequence we particularly like, for balancing the second chakra. Once you know the sequence, work on flowing from one pose to the next with as much grace and smoothness as you can. Don't worry about speed. Form is more important.

def•i•ni•tion

Surya Namaskar is the Sanskrit name for Sun Salutation, a sequence of twelve yoga poses, ideally practiced in the morning, for warming up the body and honoring the rising sun.

Sun Salutation teaches fluid strength with grace.

1. Stand in *Tadasana* (read about how to do that in Chapter 7), in bare feet with
    your feet hip-width apart. Experience stability. Bring your palms together in
    front of your heart, in prayer position. Take a deep breath to center and connect
    with something greater than yourself.

2. Inhale and bring your arms overhead, extending the spine long as you look up
    between your hands. Begin to shine your heart center up toward the ceiling, as
    you bend back slightly.

3. Exhale and bend forward at the hips, bringing your hands down toward the floor, on either side of your feet. If your hamstrings are tight and you can't touch the floor, either bend your knees so your fingers reach the floor, or put something under each hand that you can press into, such as two blocks, piles of books, or boxes.

4. Keeping your hands on the floor or other support, inhale and look up, stretching your spine forward as your chest lifts slightly, while keeping your feet and hands firmly planted. Exhale, and return to a forward bend.

5. Inhale and step your right foot back into a lunge. Keep your back thigh lifted as you bend more deeply into your front leg.

6. Exhale and step your left foot back into Plank pose, as if you were on the top end of a push-up. Inhale, and as you exhale, slowly lower yourself down to the floor with control. If you don't have the arm strength yet to lower yourself down, bring your knees to the floor before lowering your chest and head to the floor.

7. Place your hands on the mat in line with your chest, inhale and take the shoulders back, head up, and chest up. Curl into a baby back-bend. With your tailbone tucked under, extend your spine forward with every inhale. With every exhale, keep your shoulders back and soften your heart center down between the shoulder blades.

8. Exhale, bringing your head and chest back down to the mat. Curl your toes under, and with your next inhale, lift your hips off the floor. Keeping your arms straight, stretch your hips away from your shoulders. Exhale, and relax your head and neck. This is called Downward Facing Dog pose.

9. Inhale and step your right foot forward into a lunge, keeping your back leg lifting high.

10. Exhale and step forward with your left foot, returning to a forward bend, hands on the floor (or on another support) beside your feet.

11. Keeping your hands down, move your chest forward and look up as you inhale. Then exhale and bend forward again.

12. Keeping your feet firmly grounded, inhale as you sweep your arms up over your head, returning to a standing position. Bring your palms together in prayer position in line with your heart. Repeat the entire sequence as many times as you like to warm your body, and pay homage to the sun.

The Least You Need to Know

♦ The condition of your second chakra represents your passion, sexuality, fertility, creativity, and flexibility.

♦ When the second chakra is blocked, symptoms include creative blocks, infertility, sexual problems, stiffness, problems with intimate relationships, an inability to feel pleasure, and resistance to change.

♦ When the second chakra is overloaded, symptoms include over-emotionality, addictions, obsession with sex, hyper-flexibility, PMS, and excessive emotional dependence on others.

♦ You can balance the second chakra by getting professional help for addictions and relationship problems, pursuing your creativity, swimming, doing flowing yoga poses such as the Sun Salutation and other exercises such as ballet, and spending time with your immediate family.

Chapter 9

Power Chakra (*Manipura*): Your Core Self

In This Chapter

- What your Power chakra does, even without your help
- What your Power chakra represents for your body, mind, and spirit
- How to tune in to your Power chakra
- Correcting Power chakra blocks and overloads
- Using yoga for Power chakra fitness

Who are you? Your third chakra knows. Everything that distinguishes you from anybody else lives here, in your Power chakra—the seat of your individuality, personal power, and sense of self. Your third chakra is proactive. You move, act, and get things done from the third chakra, but you can also sit very still and feel who you are by focusing on this chakra. Writer Harish Johari says the third chakra "behaves like a cobra," and this is an apt metaphor for the Power chakra in several ways: the cobra can invoke fear in others, can get what it wants—but it can also harm others, or slink back down into its basket if its authority is threatened.

When your Power chakra is strong, balanced, and open, you project a confident, reliable, and trustworthy persona to the world. You exude a warmth and friendliness that others find irresistible. At its best, the third chakra projects a sense of humor and personal charisma. However, without a grounded first chakra and an emotionally balanced second chakra, the third chakra can become like a hammer or a gun, subjecting others to its power. Or if blocked, you can lose your sense of self, confidence, and ability to get anything accomplished. In other words, balancing this chakra matters a lot in terms of your ability to function in the world.

Power Chakra 101

The third chakra, Power chakra, Sun chakra, or Solar Plexus chakra, is called *Manipura* in the traditional Sanskrit. This word is usually translated as "dwelling place of the jewel," "city of jewels," or something similar, but always having to do with a jewel. This is a beautiful image, because the third chakra is where you open to abundance, prosperity, and opportunities—literally accepting the jewels of life. Harish Johari says that the body's center of gravity lies in the third chakra; so imagine a big, weighty, brilliant, priceless jewel, right below your rib cage, in the center of your solar plexus, where this chakra resides.

The third chakra is associated with the fire element because, in contrast to the first chakra's solid, grounded earthiness and the second chakra's watery, flowing movement, the third chakra projects heat and energy, as if it were the body's own inner sun. The third chakra's symbolic color is a bright sunny yellow, and the traditional lotus symbol depicting this chakra has 10 petals. The sound associated with this chakra is the seed sound *RANG*. Chanting this sound helps to activate the third chakra.

This chakra is located in your solar plexus and radiates out to encompass your stomach, pancreas, gall bladder, and liver. Your strength, as physically manifested in your muscles, is linked to the third chakra. This chakra is also associated with the middle of the back and the upper intestines.

Your Power chakra has everything to do with who you are, what you can do, and how you feel about all of that, so let's look more closely at the direct manifestation of your personal power.

When you are born, you don't understand that you and your mother are not the same being. Once you get to be two or three, however, you start to understand that you are *you*, not anyone else. You gain a sense of autonomy. This marks the beginning of your third chakra's development—but it doesn't stop there, or even in childhood.

Throughout your life, your third chakra reflects your sense of self, your ego, and who you are in your own mind.

The Power chakra (Manipura).

Understanding and accepting who you are is a lifelong process. But the third chakra can help you move more swiftly and efficiently in the right direction. A strong sense of self frees you up to get things done. It helps you to exercise your personal power in the service of building a better life for yourself. The Power chakra has a reputation for being the selfish chakra. Unfortunately, doing good things for oneself has been associated with the idea of being selfish. To truly be helpful, loving, and effective in the world, you have to be autonomous—able to function fully as a whole person, knowing and understanding yourself. Self-care and self-development is not selfish; it is essential for a healthy third chakra. You can't go through life pretending to be someone else or constantly leaning on others, and expect to succeed at it for very long. Writer, teacher, and mythology expert Joseph Campbell once wrote, "The privilege of a lifetime is being who you are." This is the birthright of the third chakra, and your birthright as well. The quest for *you* is not "selfish" in a negative way, but it is selfish … and absolutely essential.

> **Energy Unplugged**
>
> Children who grow up constantly subjected to the will of a powerful parent are likely to develop third chakra issues. If children never get to be who they are while growing up, how can they be expected to know who they are as adults? As a way to strengthen the third chakras of her own children, every night after her children are fast asleep, Betsy whispers in each of their ears "Become who you are." This ritual symbolizes Betsy's desire to support her children in whatever path they choose in life, knowing it will be *their* path, not *her* path, that she persuades them to follow.

Self-Esteem

The third chakra is not only the reflection of our sense of self, but also our opinion about ourselves. In other words, here lies your self-esteem. How do you feel about yourself? A healthy third chakra reflects a healthy appreciation of self. Too much energy here, and you may project *narcissism* and an inflated ego. Not enough energy, and you may dislike yourself, feel shame about who you are, or even feel like you don't have a personality.

def•i•ni•tion

Narcissism is a psychological term referring to a personality disorder characterized by excessive self-importance and a need for constant admiration, to such an extent that the narcissistic person is not able to love or feel empathy for others. The word comes from the Greek myth of Narcissus, who fell in love with his own reflection and died of unrequited love.

Control Issues

In addition to your identity, your third chakra is also directly related to your feelings of personal power, over yourself and others. For this reason, control issues have everything to do with the third chakra. The amount of control you exert over your own behavior, as well as the behavior of others, flows from here.

If you are compelled to control everyone and everything in your life and feel uncomfortable when you are out of control (or never let yourself get out of control), you might have an overactive third chakra. If you never feel like you have control over anything—you are a victim of circumstance, at the whim of fate, and blame others for your problems—then you might have a blocked third chakra.

Spinning Your Wheels

Betsy had a client who was a classic example of someone struggling with an overactive third chakra. This man was having difficulty maintaining close relationships. He badly wanted to find a partner, but instead found himself in many short-term relationships that went nowhere. He was extremely successful, had money, and from the outside looked like the "perfect catch."

Yet he was also arrogant and put the majority of his time into the development of his business. He would work days at a time without having contact with any friends, including the woman he was dating at the time. He thrived on stress and consistently pushed himself to achieve and find success. He had a hard time understanding why the women he dated couldn't understand his need to throw himself into his work, especially because it resulted in outward results such as money, a hot car, and expensive vacations. All his energy, however, was focused in the third chakra, taking away from his second (Passion) and fourth (Heart) chakras. The result was an unemotional man, unable to feel true empathy or intimacy with someone else, and unable to really give or receive love from a partner.

Willpower

So you can't stick with that diet? You keep procrastinating and can't finish that project? Your third chakra also reflects your willpower and your ability to follow through with your commitments. When you have a strong sense of self and personal power, you can finish what you start and do what you say (and intend). When you aren't confident in your ability to make things happen, you are less likely to have the *will* to access your own *power*. It's not surprising that those who struggle with obesity express that they have no willpower. It then becomes a vicious circle because the excess weight lowers self-esteem, which continues to keep that third chakra weak.

Moving Forward

The third chakra is also about being proactive. Strong, healthy third chakras reflect the ability to make things happen and get things done. The third chakra is the chakra of action, progress, and enacting change in the world. When you are strong here, you can move forward in your life with confidence and power.

Energy Unplugged _____

If you have trouble getting moving or have low energy, it can help to tap into the power of your third chakra through vigorous exercise. If you like to walk, step up the pace, or include short sprints. To really increase your third chakra power and energy, consider taking a class in the martial arts.

Digestive Fire

The way you process food into energy is also reflected in your third chakra. Strong third chakra people often have strong digestion, whereas people with blocked third chakras have trouble digesting many foods. Stoking your inner digestive fire through third chakra activation can not only help you feel better and get more energy from the food you eat, but can also help you achieve your ideal weight because a healthy inner fire means a healthy metabolism. You can see the effects of a healthy digestive fire in people who glow with energy. People who move sluggishly and look pale or pasty tend to have suppressed inner fire, related to a blocked third chakra.

Power Chakra Correspondences

Your Power chakra corresponds with certain colors, elements, sounds, and parts of your body, as well as parts of your life crucial to your sense of self and your ability to get things done. Check out this chart for a summary, then read on to find out how you can use your third chakra to change your life for the better.

Third Chakra	
Sanskrit name	*Manipura* (dwelling place for the jewel, city of jewels)
Element	Fire
Color	Yellow
Seed sound	*RANG*
Location	Just below the rib cage, at the solar plexus

Associated cultural phrases	"He's a man of action." "Burn the candle at both ends." "Burn the midnight oil." "Crash and burn." "More power to you!" "I have no willpower." "I need a power tie." "This will whet your appetite." "Put yourself out there."
Associated anatomy	Solar plexus, stomach, digestive organs, upper intestines, middle back, liver, pancreas, gall bladder, muscles
Associated psychological and life issues	Personal power, ego, sense of self, self-esteem, willpower, ability to get things done
Physical issues related to third chakra blockage	Sluggishness, low energy, low appetite, chronic fatigue, poor digestion, diabetes, gall bladder problems, feeling cold, stiff muscles, poor liver function, bad posture, weak middle back
Psychological issues related to third chakra blockage	Low self-esteem, lack of willpower, inability to accomplish things or follow through, unreliability, victim mentality/blaming others for problems, feeling of having no personality
Physical issues related to third chakra overloading	Hypertension, stress, ulcers, muscle spasms, insomnia due to excess energy, exercise addiction, constant hunger, physical signs related to extreme stress

continues

continued

Third Chakra	
Psychological issues related to third chakra overloading	Anger issues, control issues, obsession with power and outward signs of power such as money and possessions, inability to compromise with others, excessive competition, arrogance, lack of sensitivity, narcissism
Third chakra therapy	Aerobic exercise to increase third chakra or meditation to calm third chakra, core-strengthening exercises like sit-ups and *Pilates*, martial arts, counseling to acknowledge your inner power and potential or to develop sensitivity and respect for others

def•i•ni•tion

Pilates is a form of exercise that focuses on developing core strength while lengthening and strengthening muscles. Pilates exercises traditionally use a specific machine designed for the purpose, but can also be adapted for mat exercises, without any equipment. Pilates classes are widely available at health clubs, yoga studios, and elsewhere.

Awakening the Power Chakra

If your *Kundalini* energy is activated in your first and second chakras, then you can encourage it to rise up into your third chakra. When you awaken your Power chakra, you are likely to experience more self-confidence and ability to act, especially if you have problems getting things done. In those with overloaded Power chakras, awakening this chakra can bring your sense of self back into perspective and help you see what other people need more clearly. Awakening the Power chakra is a great way to energize and jump-start your life, increasing productivity, abundance, and self-esteem.

Anything that heats you up and strengthens your core can activate this chakra. Hot yoga styles such as Bikram yoga or core-strengthening exercises such as Pilates are great for third-chakra awakening, but so is deep relaxation for stress relief and centering, to put you back in touch with your own sense of "I." Or just go on a brisk walk or run, preferably outside on a beautiful day, but even at the gym on a treadmill if that's your only option. Sit in a sauna, or in hot moving water, submerging your solar plexus. The point is to stoke your inner fire.

To get more Power chakra energy into your environment, highlight the color yellow. Wear yellow, paint your office yellow (or just hang a yellow-dominated picture where you can see it while you work), and spend a few minutes each day in the sun. Seeing the color and feeling its warmth can help to awaken this chakra. Also include more warmth elements in your home. When was the last time you used your fireplace? Even images of fire or the sun add Power chakra energy to a room.

You can also try this exercise for awakening the Power chakra:

1. Sit on the floor, legs crossed, seat firmly planted on the floor. Feel your pelvic bones and imagine roots anchoring those bones to the earth.

2. Take several long, slow, deep breaths, and then draw your attention to the area just below your rib cage. Imagine your third chakra, a bright burning yellow circle spinning slowly, like an internal sun.

3. Imagine your third chakra radiating a yellow circle of warm, energizing light that encompasses your entire chest. Feel the warm light moving into your stomach and imagine lighting a tiny flame inside yourself, like a pilot light. Feel the warmth in your chest.

4. Take a deep breath in, and in a low resonating tone, say the word: *RANG*, holding the "A" sound (pronounced "ah;" the word rhymes with "song"). Imagine the yellow light filling your entire body with slow, steady beams of inner sunlight.

5. Continue to breathe and let the warm beams fill you with a feeling of benevolent power and confidence, radiating from your third chakra, as long as you like.

Aligning the Power Chakra

Let the power of the sun help pull your Power chakra into alignment with this exercise:

1. Stand outside in the sun, on a sunny day. Plant your feet firmly on the ground. Hold your arms out about a foot away from the sides of your body and rotate your palms to face up. Close your eyes and lift your face to the sun.

2. Imagine your third chakra, just below your rib cage, and try to feel it spinning. Feel the rays of the sun beaming straight down into the crown of your head, and imagine them flowing down through your spine to merge with your Power chakra.

3. Imagine your Power chakra spinning more quickly, then beaming yellow sun energy back up through the crown of your head, to merge with the sun's energy.

4. Lift your arms straight up overhead and imagine the yellow light pulsing up and down, radiating to the sun and back again. Your chakra should now be aligned.

Blocks in the Power Chakra

Our culture certainly values power. We see control as a positive quality and being out-of-control as a distinctly negative quality. We prize people who achieve, make things happen, and radiate personal charisma, even if they use that charisma to control others in order to get ahead.

In many ways, power *is* a positive thing, though even the more idealistic among us tend to associate it across the board with greed. To feel powerless is certainly not healthy. Feeling powerful, knowing you can control your own destiny and influence the events of your own life, is a very good thing. Power only turns negative when we use it against others or lack the sensitivity to understand how our actions affect those around us.

But if you have a blocked power chakra, carelessly wielding your power is the least of your problems. You tend to feel powerless and out-of-control. A blocked Power chakra often results in low self-esteem and self-destructive behaviors that can lead to victimization by others. If you let other people take advantage of you, you can almost guarantee that they will (especially those people with overloaded third chakras!).

Blocked Chakra Health Issues

Third chakra issues usually relate to digestion and poor posture. Conditions like diabetes, hypoglycemia, or problems in the gall bladder and liver may be related to the third chakra. So is a chronic lack of energy, such as chronic fatigue syndrome or fibromyalgia. People with blocked third chakras also appear collapsed in the middle. Their abdominal and/or lower back muscles tend to be weak and they slump, instead of standing tall and radiating power. They don't feel that power, so they can't send it out—and the result is an inability to even maintain the basic core structure of the body.

Blocked Chakra Psychological Issues

People with blocked third chakras tend to put themselves down a lot, blame other people for their problems, and complain of low energy. At the heart of a third chakra block is a weak sense of "I." Blocked third chakra people may seem to others to have very little personality, and indeed, that's often how they feel. They often constrict their feelings, and refuse to let others see how they really feel. The third chakra reflects your sense of yourself, and if you don't have a clear sense of who you are, or you don't like who you are and try to disengage from it, all the energy that should be channeled into the practice of engaging with the world dissipates. .

> **Energy Unplugged** _____
>
> Temporary third chakra blocks can sometimes be caused by a professional setback. Many of us tend to associate at a very deep level with the work we do. When that work is questioned or criticized, we take it very personally. If you are experiencing a problem at your job, it is very important to separate that problem from your sense of personal worth. If you don't, you can set yourself up for a continued downward spiral of failure in your work, which continues to feed your degrading sense of self, until you aren't able to fix the problem. Instead, if you let work be work and you be you, then you will be more objective about the situation and better able to address the problem, whatever it is, in a more rational (and powerful) way.

Healing a Blocked Third Chakra

To unblock your third chakra, think about heating your body and strengthening your core. Some great ways to do that, and some other ideas for healing your blocked Power chakra, include:

- Exercising until you sweat. Running—even short sprints—is a great third chakra exercise.

- Sitting in a sauna or a steam room.

- Doing hot yoga, such as Bikram yoga.

- Taking a Pilates class.

- Eating yellow foods, especially when they are spicy or have the strong flavors of ginger, cinnamon, turmeric, and curry.

- Engaging in positive self-talk. Tell yourself you are strong, capable, and active. Saying things repeatedly to yourself can help you begin to believe them.

♦ Employing mantras such as: *I am strong and powerful. I believe in and celebrate myself. I open to the prosperity and abundance in the universe. I can accomplish and complete anything I want to do.*

♦ Finding a task you can finish, that will make even a small difference in your environment, such as cleaning out a drawer, loading the dishwasher, or making your bed. Go do it, and don't stop until you are finished.

♦ Spending time with a friend who genuinely values you and is good at letting you know it (but we're not talking about flattery here, remember!).

♦ Getting counseling for self-esteem issues.

Energy Unplugged

An easy way to tune up your third chakra is to listen to your own inner voice. What messages do you tell yourself throughout the day? Do these messages build you up or tear you down? If you are always criticizing yourself for your failures rather than patting yourself on the back for your successes, you are encouraging the block in your third chakra. Work on purposefully stuffing a sock in that negative voice and focusing on your strengths. Let yourself talk to yourself about all your great qualities—because you have a lot of them!

Overloading in the Power Chakra

Overloaded Power chakras are easy to recognize. These are the loud, steal-all-the-attention-in-the-room, do-it-my-way, I-have-to-have-the-last-word people. Maybe this is you, but even if it isn't, you probably know people like this. An overloaded third chakra makes you arrogant and self-centered. You always think you are right, and people who don't agree with you don't just have different opinions. They are *wrong*.

If you lived all alone in the world, an overloaded third chakra might not be much of a problem. However, as long as you have to get along with other people—feeling empathy from your second chakra and genuine love and compassion from your Heart chakra—an overloaded third chakra will thwart your attempts at satisfactory relationships, not to mention spiritual progress. If you seek access to a higher power, you'll have a lot of trouble seeing around your own inflated ego.

Overloaded Chakra Health Issues

Overloaded third chakra people tend to have very high stress, and all the physical problems that go along with that, such as hypertension, tight muscles, and ulcers. Although chronic fatigue is typical of people with blocked third chakras, overloaded third chakra people tend to be so keyed up all the time that at some point, their bodies can't take it anymore and they collapse from exhaustion. These are the people admitted to the emergency room because they think they are having a heart attack, when in actuality they are having severe indigestion, possible panic attacks, and total exhaustion. Overloaded third chakra people also have a tendency to overuse pain medications and sedatives, in a misguided attempt to calm down. It's hard work carrying around a gigantic ego. Those things are heavy!

Energy Unplugged

Got stress? Meditation is an excellent way to begin practicing stress relief. Try sitting in a comfortable position and tuning in to your immediate environment or breath for just five quiet minutes. No phone, no computer, no sound other than soothing music, if that helps to relax you. When thoughts come to mind, look at them as if they belonged to someone else, then let them go. You may need to let go of a thousand thoughts over the course of five minutes, and this is perfectly okay and normal. The point is to keep letting thoughts go rather than letting them carry you away. Keep returning to the rhythm of your breathing or the sound of the music in the room. The more you practice, the better you will get. Meditation gives your busy mind a break, which is crucial for people who tend to be overloaded in the third chakra.

Overloaded Chakra Lifestyle Issues

Overloaded third chakra people can come across not only as arrogant but also as just plain mean, especially to people who are particularly sensitive (overloaded in the second chakra). Overloaded Power chakra people just can't understand why people do things other than their way, which is obviously the right way. When the world doesn't oblige them, they can become snappy, aggressive, and even violent. If you've ever seen an adult throw a temper tantrum, you can bet an overloaded third chakra is involved.

Overloaded third chakra people tend to be very successful and are good at acquiring all the trappings of success and power. They are also prone to losing it all in one fell swoop, however, because they take risks and don't usually consider other points of view. This can be a lonely way to live, so balancing that third chakra is well worth the effort.

Healing an Overloaded Power Chakra

Healing an overloaded Passion chakra means draining out some of that excessive "all-about-me" energy, to make room for other kinds of energy, like grounding energy, compassion, and love. Remember, personal power is great, as long as it doesn't take over and exercise its power at the expense of others. Balance is best. Try these strategies:

- Practice deep relaxation techniques, such as meditation or *Savasana* (see Chapter 7).

- Aerobic exercise, such as running or working out at the gym, to drain off aggressive energy.

- Practice deep breathing exercises. Take long, slow, deep breaths, filling up your lungs completely, then exhaling completely. Try inhaling to the count of five and exhaling to the count of ten, increasing these intervals with practice.

- Engage in noncompetitive activities, or activities that force you to work with others.

- Slow down. Practice eating, walking, even working in a slower and more measured way.

- Hone your listening skills. Practice hearing what other people are saying. Try posing the question to yourself: "What if they really are right and I'm wrong?" It's not the end of the world if that turns out to be true. In fact, it's good for you, like eating vegetables … or humble pie!

- Get counseling to learn to increase your sensitivity toward others and for anger management issues.

Spinning Your Wheels

When you first begin practicing the Warrior poses, it is not uncommon to feel fears and anxieties arise in these challenging poses. Warrior II was Betsy's least favorite pose for years. Despite a strong practice, she always experienced an irrational fear that her legs wouldn't be able to support her. As her teacher kept the class in this pose, Betsy would routinely feel panicky, and her mind would begin to race with fears of collapsing. It wasn't until she worked with a Phoenix Rising Sun yoga therapist, that she began to connect her personal struggle with stepping into her own potential and power with her difficulty in Warrior II pose. As she worked on increasing the fire in her third chakra, burned through old and limiting fears, began to believe in herself, and took some risks in her life that forced her to be the powerful woman she is, Warrior II suddenly become easier. She now joyfully holds Warrior II with steadfastness, inner fortitude, and a calm mind.

Yoga Poses to Balance the Power Chakra

The best yoga poses for balancing both blocked and overloaded Power chakras are those poses that help you to feel powerful but balanced, and those poses that strengthen your core. The Warrior series is ideal for this purpose. So is Boat pose, which not only builds core strength but also teaches you balance from the inside out.

Warrior I (*Virabhadrasana I*)

The first Warrior pose.

1. Stand in *Tadasana* (as described in Chapter 7) in bare feet, with your feet hip-width apart. Experience stability. Take a deep breath and allow the strength of something greater to support you as you prepare to become a warrior.

2. Inhale and step or jump your feet about 3 to 4 feet apart. Turn your left foot in a little, and open your right leg 90 degrees to the front of your yoga mat. Square your hips to face the front of your mat. If you feel unsteady, you can walk your left foot more to the edge of your mat to create a wider base from which to work.

3. Firm your muscles and hug your shins toward each other. Keeping your left leg straight, exhale and bend your right leg into a square. Your right knee should track to the little toe side of your right foot.

4. Inhale and stretch your arms up toward the ceiling. Your upper arms should be on either side of your ears.

5. Take your upper inner groins back and apart. Maintaining the thighs back now, lengthen the tailbone down toward your heels as you lunge deeper into the front leg. Press your feet firmly into the mat, sending energy from the core of your pelvis down into the earth.

6. Inhale and straighten your front leg. Turn your feet to be parallel, then step or jump your feet back together. Repeat on the other side.

Warrior II (*Virabhadrasana II*)

The second warrior pose.

Correct   Arched   Flat

1. Stand in *Tadasana* (as described in Chapter 7) in bare feet, with your feet hip-width apart. Experience stability. Take a deep breath and allow the strength of something greater to support you as you prepare to become a warrior.

2. Inhale and step or jump your feet about 3 to 4 feet apart. Turn your left foot in a little, and open your right leg 90 degrees to the front of your mat. Your right foot should be directly in line with the arch of your left foot. Raise your arms to the side. Your ankles should be in line with your wrists.

3. Firm your muscles and hug your shins toward each other. Keeping your left leg straight, exhale and bend your right leg into a square, so your knee is directly over your ankle. Your right knee should track to the little toe side of your right foot. Turn your head to gaze out over your right hand.

4. Concentrate on feeling power in your legs. Rely on your breath to support you in this challenging pose. With every inhale, elongate your spine; with every exhale, ground down into your legs as you lunge more deeply into your right leg.

5. Inhale and straighten your bent leg. Step or jump your feet back together. Repeat on the other side.

Boat Pose *(Navasana)*

Practicing boat pose with a partner.

1. Sit on the floor and stretch your legs straight out in front of you.

2. Keeping your body straight and your core muscles firm, exhale and lean back, raising your legs to 60 degrees and lowering the trunk by 30 degrees. Balance on the front of the buttock bones. Extend energy out through the legs, keeping the feet flexed.

3. Raise the arms to shoulder level, palms facing each other, and stretch the arms long. Breathe evenly and try to balance for as long as you can.

4. Come down slowly.

The Least You Need to Know

- The condition of your third chakra represents your sense of self, ego, self-esteem, willpower, and ability to get things done.

- When the third chakra is blocked, symptoms include low self-esteem, sluggishness, victim mentality, low energy, chronic fatigue, weak core muscles, slow digestion, poor appetite, and problems with the pancreas, gall bladder, and liver.

- When the third chakra is overloaded, symptoms include aggressiveness, arrogance, too much energy, irritability, violence, ambitiousness at the expense of others, an inability to feel empathy, high stress, hypertension, muscle spasms, and overuse of painkillers or sedatives.

- You can balance the third chakra by working up a sweat, doing hot yoga and other heating exercises, sitting in a sauna or steam room, spending time in the sun, listening to others, slowing down, and strengthening the muscles of your core.

Chapter 10

Heart Chakra (*Anahata*): Love Is Everything

In This Chapter

- ◆ What your Heart chakra does, even without your help
- ◆ What your Heart chakra represents for your body, mind, and spirit
- ◆ How to tune in to your Heart chakra
- ◆ Correcting Heart chakra blocks and overloads
- ◆ Using yoga for Heart chakra fitness

Do we have to tell you that your fourth chakra is all about love? Of course it is. This is your Heart chakra, the place where loving energy pours out of you to wash over the world and make life better. Your bonds to other human beings, your sense of caring and compassion, your altruism, your urge to give to others, and, just as importantly, your ability to love, cherish, and take care of yourself all start here.

Plus, the Heart chakra is the center chakra, halfway between the three lower, earthier, and more physical chakras and the three higher, more cerebral and spiritual chakras. The Heart chakra is the fulcrum, where you find balance between Earth and heaven and between body and mind. Love holds it all together and makes you human. In other words, this chakra is a V.I.C. (very important chakra!).

When your Heart chakra is strong, balanced, and open, you know how to love and give to others freely, but you also know how to love and take care of yourself. When the Heart chakra is blocked, however, you may feel cut off from your connection to others. An overloaded Heart chakra, by contrast, is linked to giving *too* much, at the expense of your physical and emotional health. Let's explore the Heart chakra in more depth, so you can get your center of balance *back* into balance and celebrate what might just be the very best quality of human beings: the ability to love.

Heart Chakra 101

The fourth chakra, also sometimes called the Heart, Love, or Air chakra, is called *Anahata* in the traditional Sanskrit. This word can be translated as "unstruck" or "intact." Some scholars call this chakra the "place of the unstruck sound," because the heart sings without having to be played (we think that's such a nice way to think about the Heart chakra).

The fourth chakra is associated with the air element, perhaps because you breathe from here. This is the realm not only of the heart but of the lungs—in fact, the entire cardiovascular system. Life force energy moves in and out from here. You could think of your fourth chakra as your very own Grand Central Station. The fourth chakra's symbolic color is green and the traditional lotus symbol depicting this chakra has 12 petals. The sound associated with this chakra is the seed sound *YANG*. Chanting this sound helps to activate the fourth chakra.

We bet you can guess where this chakra is located—right behind your heart, radiating in and around your heart, lungs, chest, and even out to your shoulders, down your arms, and into your hands. Other physical structures associated with the fourth chakra are your thymus gland and your cardiac nerve plexus. For women, the breasts are also the realm of the fourth chakra.

Balance

At the heart of the Heart chakra is the notion of balance. As we mentioned earlier, the Heart chakra sits squarely between the three lower chakras and the three higher chakras. Your first, second, and third chakras have everything to do with the physical body, whereas the fifth, sixth, and seventh chakras are more about intuition, the mind, and the spirit. The Heart chakra helps these two halves of you speak to each other and act, not out of pure physical instinct or completely in-your-head braininess, but with active love and compassion.

The Heart chakra (Anahata).

Finding balance, strength, and openness in your fourth chakra will transform your life into one of balance, strength, and open-heartedness.

Energy Unplugged _____

Children who don't feel loved or who feel their love is rejected by a parent or a sibling often develop blocked Heart chakras. They fear more rejection so they close down this sensitive chakra and refuse to make themselves vulnerable. Sometimes, children grow up with an opposite reaction: an overloaded Heart chakra so focused on giving to others in an effort to make up for a lack of love and attention in their life that they never learn how to take care of themselves or how to receive love. Consider how your family handled issues of love, compassion, and giving to others, as well as caring for themselves. Are you repeating or reflecting those patterns in your adult life?

Love Fest

Love. It makes the world go around. It's what the world needs. It's the answer. Our culture is obsessed with love, as is obvious by the music we create and play over and over again, by the movies and television shows we watch, by the stories that move us to tears, even by our entire value system, which champions such notions as marriage, true love, soul mates, love at first sight, and romance.

We have a huge capacity to love—so huge that we extend that love beyond our own species. We love our dogs, our cats, our birds, even our fish. We love our plants. We love the earth. We love mountains and starry skies and flowers. In other words, *we love*. And it all comes out of the fourth chakra.

When we lose love, when our hearts are broken, we can literally feel it in our fourth chakra. That feeling of pain, grief, a shattered heart, is very real, even if a doctor couldn't pinpoint it with a diagnostic test. If you've ever had your heart broken, you know what we mean.

Fortunately, the fourth chakra is also an expert healer.

Healing Power

The fourth chakra energy naturally flows not only around your heart and lungs but also down your arms and out the palms of your hands. This means that when this chakra is strong and energized, your hands actually have healing power. This healing may be subtle, but it is very real. Think about how a mother's loving touch on her child's wounded knee seems to make everything better. You can even use this natural healing ability on yourself to cycle your own loving energy back through your body. This is one of the best ways to love yourself and make yourself strong, healthy, vibrant, and able to love others well.

You can use your own healing energy to help speed the healing of your aches, pains, strains, sprains, and even your emotional pain, from a bruised ego to a broken heart. Just try this healing meditation:

- Sit comfortably anywhere. Close your eyes. Visualize your heart chakra as an emerald-green wheel of light spinning around your heart.

- Breathe deeply and imagine the light growing brighter and more vibrant. Imagine the wheel spinning faster. Imagine the chakra getting larger and more brilliant.

- Visualize that green light now, and picture it flowing out from the sides of the chakra, up through your shoulders, down your arms, and out your palms.

- Bring your palms about 2 inches apart and try to feel the energy between them. Continue to visualize that heart energy flowing, like an eternal spring, from out of your heart chakra, down your arms and out your hands.

- Touch your palms together and feel the healing energy moving in a two-directional circle, from your heart, down each arm, and back up each opposite arm at the same time.

- Now, put your palms onto any part of your body that hurts. Imagine the green light filled with tiny sparks of healing energy, pouring into the spot and knitting and mending everything back together, healing and connecting tissues and strengthening bones and joints, freeing internal energy to move where it needs to go.

- Stay like this, with your palms on the hurt area, for as long as you like. Repeat several times each day, if possible.

Spinning Your Wheels

Betsy sees so many people in treatment with fourth chakra heart issues! She believes this is the chakra we shut down most often, as a means of protecting ourselves. Yet what starts out as self-preservation often turns into isolation and disconnection from those relationships that we are wired to need in our lives.

Your Compassion Center

The fourth chakra is not only about love, but also about other impulses that are born out of love, especially compassion. To live a life of loving kindness and compassion toward others is to live a life with the fourth chakra wide open. Our culture admires people who feel compassion for others and act on that compassion. We act on our compassion in many ways, from formalized expression such as joining the Peace Corps or volunteering for a charity, to quieter ways, like being a good listener for a friend, being open to family members who need help, and even feeling compassion for ourselves and our own needs.

But compassion has a dark side, too. Some people are so open and overloaded in their fourth chakras that compassion for others takes over their lives. They dedicate all their energies to helping others, while completely neglecting their own needs. A balanced fourth chakra can feel compassion for others while also feeling compassion for the self.

Spinning Your Wheels _____

A recent client came to Betsy for treatment because she was dissatisfied with her marriage. She had been married for about three years, and she felt that her husband didn't communicate his feelings to her enough. She also didn't feel like he heard her when she was speaking. She feared their relationship was doomed, and had already begun to shut herself off emotionally from her husband. Betsy soon learned that this woman came from a supportive and nurturing home where open and loving communication was the norm. Her parents were still married after 35 years, and had a very loving relationship. In fact, the woman had never seen her parents fight or even be cross with one another.

While it might seem like such an upbringing would be a recipe for a healthy fourth chakra, the problem was that this woman had very specific expectations for her own marriage. When it didn't look like her parents' marriage, she assumed something was terribly wrong and it was destined to fail. Through their work together, focusing on the fourth chakra, Betsy helped this woman to re-open her heart and see that she and her husband were not her parents. They had to forge their own way through love, rather than turning into a mirror image of the woman's past. She also realized that she could not compare her 3-year marriage with her parents' 35-year relationship. The woman expressed great relief. Now she understands that fighting doesn't have to mean divorce, and that in letting go of her colossal expectations, she can embrace what love is for *her.*

Let's Talk About *You*

You've probably heard the old saying that you can't love others until you love yourself. That's not exactly true. You *can* love others without loving yourself, but it will be a needy, clingy, immature love compared to love that comes from an autonomous and full heart. Your fourth chakra reflects your self-love in the same way it reflects your ability to give love and receive love from others.

You are in a primary relationship with yourself. As you treat others, so you should treat yourself, and vice versa. Do you speak to yourself with the same compassion and care that you use to speak to your loved ones? Most people admit that they are much more cruel and judgmental toward themselves. Without self-love, self-care, self-nurturing, and compassion for your own needs and desires, your fourth chakra will never be completely open and vibrantly healthy.

What Goes Out Must Come In

The fourth chakra gets a lot of press for being all about loving others, but a healthy fourth chakra can also receive love *from* others. Think of the fourth chakra not as a waterfall but as the entire water cycle.

There is an old Hindu legend that Shiva and Shakti, the primordial God and Goddess, make love constantly on a mountaintop. Their passion is so intense that it melts the snow, which runs down the mountain and becomes the sacred Ganges River. But the story doesn't stop there. That river water evaporates in the intense heat, forms clouds, floats over the mountain, and snows down again onto the loving couple, and the cycle starts all over again. That's how your fourth chakra should work: your love flows outward, but comes back to you, too.

> **Energy Unplugged**
>
> Physically opening your Heart chakra can actually make more room to get Heart chakra energy flowing in a healthier way. If you usually slump and hold your shoulders and head forward, you are actually physically sheltering your heart chakra. To get more open, pull your shoulders back, look up, and imagine lifting your heart toward the sky. Yoga back-bending poses like the ones at the end of this chapter are a great way to open the heart, but even a good stretch that expands the chest and pulls your shoulders back can make a difference.

Girl Talk

Gentlemen, feel free to skip this section. Ladies, let's talk about The Girls. The Twins. The Two Sisters. That's right, we mean your breasts.

Yes, the fourth chakra has everything to do with this most female of female body parts. Your breasts literally transmit love to your baby by feeding the most perfect food, but even if you've never breastfed a baby, your breasts are all about love. Your sense of womanhood is all tied up in your breasts, and woven into your fourth chakra.

We would be remiss if we didn't mention breast cancer, as millions of women each year are diagnosed with it. Although researchers understand that genetics, lifestyle, diet, and hormones put women at risk for it, it is nearly impossible to pinpoint why certain people get it and others do not. From an energetic perspective based upon chakra theory, breast cancer is likely related to an imbalance in the fourth chakra. Breasts represent love and nurturing. If disease shows up at the Heart chakra, it may be important to ask yourself if you are nurturing others at the expense of your own self-care. Ask yourself what you want and need. Disease comes into our lives to help us understand ourselves more deeply and seek balance.

You can open your Heart chakra by improving your posture. Lift your heart!

Your breasts are particularly sensitive to how well you love yourself, and how well you receive love. Breasts are, by their very nature, all about giving, so if they don't receive love in return, you feel it. Love yourself, love your female nature, take care of yourself, and honor yourself for the goddess that you really are, and you'll be taking care of your breasts, too.

Spinning Your Wheels

Just before starting this book, Betsy gave birth to a beautiful baby boy—her second. Everything was going well until Betsy developed a nasty case of mastitis—an infection of the milk ducts in the breast that is characterized by pain, fever, and flu-like symptoms. Betsy believes that her mastitis was directly linked to an overflowing amount of love, nourishment, and protection which she was giving away, not only to her new infant but to her three-year-old son, and to her fledgling yoga studio (her other baby). Betsy was focused so intensely on the needs of others that she was doing absolutely nothing for herself in terms of rest and self-care. Her fourth chakra was so wide open that her body went into emergency alert mode. Voilà—mastitis. Betsy didn't just get mastitis once, but twice, when she didn't get the message the first time. When she finally realized she needed to drop some of her less important responsibilities (such as those at the yoga studio) and began to say "no" to requests from other people, and when she sent her three-year-old for a visit with his Grandma and focused on nothing but feeding her baby, resting, and nourishing herself, she finally got … and stayed … better. Lesson learned.

Heart Chakra Correspondences

Your Heart chakra corresponds with so many aspects of your life because humans live with love so central to their consciousness. Consider the associations in the following chart and consider how your Heart chakra fits into who you are.

Fourth Chakra	
Sanskrit name	*Anahata* (unstruck, intact, dwelling place of the unstruck sound)
Element	Air
Color	Green
Seed sound	*YANG*
Location	Behind the heart
Associated cultural phrases	"Love makes the world go 'round." "All you need is love." "Love is the answer." "My heart is broken." "Bleeding-heart."

continues

continued

Fourth Chakra	
Associated anatomy	Heart, lungs, shoulders, arms, chest, breasts, thymus gland, cardiac nerve plexus
Associated psychological and life issues	Giving and receiving love, balance, healing, charity, compassion, self-love
Physical issues related to fourth chakra blockage	Heart problems related to blockage (angina, heart disease, heart attack); lung and breathing problems (asthma, shortness of breath, pleurisy, emphysema); pain in the chest, shoulders, or arms; immune system suppression; depression
Psychological issues related to fourth chakra blockage	Withdrawal from intimate relationships, coldness, intolerance, irritability and impatience, being overly critical of others, lack of compassion and empathy for others, chronic relationship failure
Physical issues related to fourth chakra overload	Enlarged heart, low blood pressure, depression, exhaustion, breast problems (breast cancer, mastitis, benign lumps)
Psychological issues related to fourth chakra overload	Constantly putting needs of others above yourself, martyr complex, burn-out, codependency in relationships, clinginess, self-neglect, jealousy, chronic relationship failures
Fourth chakra therapy	Deep breathing and breathing exercises; eating lots of fruits and vegetables; back-bends; volunteering and charity work (for blockages); spending more time with animals; spending more time with children; counseling or therapy to help with relationship issues, grief/loss issues, and/or self-esteem and self-care issues

Awakening the Heart Chakra

When *Kundalini* energy is free to move through your fourth chakra, you've accomplished something important: connecting your body and mind in a powerful way. When you awaken your Heart chakra, you are likely to experience strong feelings of love and compassion, not only for the people you already know you love, but for all living things—people, animals, the natural world. No, you won't become some flaky, disconnected, head-in-the-clouds love guru. We promise. But you will become more loving, and be able to both feel and express your loving energy in a more meaningful way.

Awakening the Heart chakra also means you'll feel more comfortable being loved, and that's a big step for some people. And finally, you'll be better at loving yourself. You might even begin to understand why that is so important.

Anything that physically or metaphorically opens your heart and chest area will help to awaken your Heart chakra. The other key: filling up with air. Deep breathing and yogic *pranayama* exercises are essential for Heart chakra activation. Remember, this chakra's symbolic element is air, and breath is the aspect of the air element that you can control.

To get more Heart chakra energy into your environment, emphasize the color green. Wear green, paint your family room green, or put green plants around the house. Just seeing the color can help to awaken this chakra. Also include more air elements in your home, such as fans to move air, and wind chimes and mobiles to produce sound and movement when the air moves. Open the windows whenever you can, to get fresh air moving through your home.

You can also try this exercise for awakening the Heart chakra:

1. Sit on the floor, legs crossed, seat on a pillow or a folded blanket. Feel your pelvic bones and imagine roots anchoring those bones to the earth. Place your hands slightly behind you and move your shoulders back to open your chest.

2. Take several long, slow, deep breaths, and then draw your attention to the area just behind your heart. Imagine your fourth chakra, a brilliant, emerald-green circle spinning slowly.

3. Imagine your chakra radiating a green circle of brilliant light that encompasses your entire chest. Feel the warmth melting your heart, so that all the hardness falls away and you feel open and radiating with love.

4. Take a deep breath in and in a low resonating tone, say the word: *YANG*, holding the "A" sound (pronounced "ah;" the word rhymes with "song"). Imagine the green light filling your entire body with slow, steady pulses, like a heartbeat.

5. Continue to breathe and let the warm waves of love and compassion continue to radiate from your fourth chakra, as long as you like.

Aligning the Heart Chakra

Set your heart right, and all your other chakras above and below will get pulled into line as love moves both up and down from this central chakra. To get your Heart chakra properly aligned, try this exercise:

1. Stand in Mountain pose, with your feet about hip-width apart, arms at your sides.

2. Imagine your fourth chakra just behind your heart, and try to feel it spinning and getting warmer. Imagine your heart softening.

3. Visualize a strong green cord moving straight up out of your Heart chakra, up through the crown of your head, filling your entire upper body with healing energy. Now, visualize this strong green cord of healing energy shooting straight down from your heart, down through your third, second, and first chakras and down into the earth. Imagine the entire cord filling your body with healing energy as it beams straight up and straight down.

4. Lift your arms straight up overhead and imagine the green light flowing up and down, radiating to the center of the earth and all the way to the sky. Your chakra should now be aligned.

Blocks in the Heart Chakra

So many people have Heart chakra blocks! We believe many things can cause Heart chakra blockages, from childhood all the way up to what happened to you five minutes ago. Because this is such an important, central chakra, however, it is essential to keep the heart unblocked. For many people, unblocking the Heart chakra may be a daily priority. When your Heart chakra flows freely after being blocked, your life will change because you will see the entire world—the universe, and everybody and everything in it—in an entirely new way. You will begin to understand what it means to *love*, even when love is difficult.

To have an open heart is to fulfill your destiny as a sentient being. When the Heart chakra is blocked, you withdraw from people and from real connection. You judge others and yourself harshly. You get irritated and you run from intimacy. Maybe you have commitment issues, or even rage issues. You might be lonely, but at least you are autonomous, and strong. Or, at least, that's what you tell yourself.

But in reality, you are lonely because a blocked Heart chakra is characterized by deep spiritual longing. Not only does a blocked Heart chakra keep you from connecting with other people, but it also blocks the connection between your body and your mind. It may even block your connection with something larger, with spirit, with God, with the power of the universe.

Many people fall into the habit of systematically keeping their Heart chakra blocked. They learn this pattern when they get their hearts broken and don't want to feel that pain again. This could have happened as a child or as an adult, after profound loss, a failed relationship, or getting hurt by anyone for any reason.

But that's not your destiny. Your Heart chakra knows (and that means *you* know) that what is easiest is not always what is best.

Blocked Chakra Health Issues

Fourth chakra health issues have everything to do with your heart, lungs, and chest. When your Heart chakra is blocked, your heart can physically become blocked, resulting in heart disease, clogged arteries, angina (chest pain), and heart attack. (Of course, not everyone with heart disease has a blocked heart chakra. This can be caused by many other environmental and genetic factors.) A blocked Heart chakra can also contribute to blocked breathing passages, asthma, and shallow breathing, as well as lung pain.

Blocked Heart chakra types can also experience depression, because of the loneliness and isolation they maintain. You can see a blocked Heart chakra in someone with a sunken chest or a hunched upper back. Instead of leading with the heart, the body is literally protecting the Heart chakra by coiling forward.

Blocked Chakra Psychological Issues

When the Heart chakra is blocked, there are multiple psychological implications. Most obviously, people with blocked Heart chakras have problems relating to other people, commitment issues, and relationship problems. The people who are afraid to get married have blocked Heart chakras, while the people who are overloaded in their

Heart chakras may find themselves in dysfunctional codependent relationships where they are so enmeshed with their partner that they lose all sense of individuality and independence.

Heart chakra blockages also reflect a judgmental attitude. These are the people who are so critical of others (and most of all, of themselves) that every fault in someone becomes an obstacle to a relationship. No one is ever quite good enough—although in reality, what people with blocked Heart chakras are actually feeling is that *they* aren't good enough, or deserving enough, to ever experience love.

> **Energy Unplugged**
>
> When someone breaks your heart, it is very important to nurture your fourth chakra back to health again. It may need to close down for a while, and that's fine. Be patient with yourself, and most of all, take care of yourself. When you nurture and attend to your own needs, the love you give to yourself will help coax your fourth chakra open again. Remember, the fourth chakra is the healing chakra. Only when it opens again can you truly experience self-healing.

Healing a Blocked Fourth Chakra

To heal and strengthen a blocked Heart chakra, Betsy encourages her clients to care for themselves. You can't control how or whether others love you, but you can control how and whether you love yourself. She reminds her clients that the most important relationship one will ever have is the relationship with oneself. This means you better put some effort into this relationship, because it is literally the only relationship you are guaranteed to have up to your dying day. If you are always pulling away from others, look first into your own heart. Are you pulling away from yourself? Heal your fear of self-love first, and loving others, as well as accepting love from others, will happen automatically. If you don't know how to do this, a therapist can help.

The fourth chakra also heals and opens when you practice loving things that are easier to love than human adults. Animals—especially companion animals like dogs and cats, children, even nature can soften and open your heart when it has closed down. If you don't have pets or children, take some time to volunteer at an animal shelter or a school. Spend more time outside, in direct contact with nature. Walk in the park or hike in a natural area. All these activities can help to fill up your heart so that it opens again.

Also focus on your breath. Anything that gets your breath moving will help to open your heart. Try some of these activities to open a blocked Heart chakra:

- Practice deep breathing and the yoga breathing exercises called *pranayama* (like the one later in this chapter called *Nadi Shodhana*).

- Eat green foods like salads, spinach, kale, collard greens, Swiss chard, green beans, artichokes, and sweet peas.

- Reach out to help others in need, through volunteer work or through simple, kindly gestures to strangers.

- Get up in the air. Climb a tree. Ride a Ferris wheel. Hike up a mountain, or just go up on a roof and take in the view.

- Hug someone who loves you. You don't have to say a word.

- Spend time with children, preferably outside.

- Meditate on your loving feelings for someone. Dedicate your day to someone you love.

- Make a list of all your own good qualities. If you are having trouble, ask someone who loves you to help.

- Exercise, especially anything that increases your breathing, such as brisk walking, running, or dancing.

- Engage in Anusara yoga. This form of yoga literally means "flowing with grace, following your heart." Anusara is a heart-oriented style of yoga that combines attention to alignment and a life-affirming philosophy. Every Anusara class focuses on a heart-opening theme.

- Recite these mantras: *I love and nourish myself. I deserve love. It's okay to love. I will open my heart and allow others to love me. The world is a better place because I love.*

Energy Unplugged

An easy way to tune up your fourth chakra is to pay attention to the ways other people express love, not only to you but also to others in their lives. How do other people show love to their partners, to their children, to their friends, and even to their pets? Watch and you might learn something. You can even copy some of their words or gestures, to try them on for size. Some people are very good at loving.

Overload in the Heart Chakra

Maybe you don't have any problem loving others. Maybe your problem is that you love *too much*. But wait. Is that really possible? Can there be too much love in the world?

The problem with an overloaded Heart chakra is not that you have too much love, but that you are out of balance. You let your Heart chakra dominate your other chakras, at their expense. A full, open, loving Heart chakra is a wonderful quality, but if your Power (below) and Truth (above) chakras atrophy because your Heart chakra is so huge, you can lose a sense of who you are and what is really best for you.

People with overloaded Heart chakras are those people who give and give and give until they burn out—or suffer from immune system collapse or heart failure. Can you say *martyr complex?* These people might be trying desperately to gain the love of others—perhaps because they didn't receive enough as children—so much so that they go overboard. They often end up in codependent relationships or are clingy and smothering to their partners and/or children.

def•i•ni•tion

Martyr complex is a psychological term referring to someone who suffers on purpose, often in the name of helping or serving someone else, suffering for love, or suffering for a cause, at the expense of personal needs or desires. This type of person often becomes resentful because the love they shower on others isn't returned to them in the way they want.

Overloaded Chakra Health Issues

Physical signs of an overloaded fourth chakra include low blood pressure, an enlarged heart, exhaustion, depression, and self-neglect. Women with overloaded Heart chakras may develop breast problems, such as benign cysts, breast pain, sometimes even cancer, as they keep pouring out love without saving some of that love for themselves. People with overloaded Heart chakras sometimes stand with their chests forward, but not in the overpowering way that overloaded third-chakra people lead with their solar plexus. Instead, this kind of chest-forward stance looks more barrel-chested and vulnerable, with the head pulled back, almost as if they are physically offering their hearts out to anyone.

> (!!!) **Wake-Up Call** _____
>
> In many relationships, one person gives much more than they receive, and the other person receives much more than they give. Considering that the fourth chakra is the chakra of balance, this is definitely a fourth chakra–related problem. Consider whether you give more than you get in your relationship, or whether you take more than you give. Either way, you aren't getting everything you could because your relationship is unbalanced. What could you do to shift the power more toward the fulcrum? Ironically, sometimes the best way to get more is actually to give more. Try meditating on that with your fourth chakra open.

Overloaded Chakra Psychological Issues

Overloaded fourth chakras result in big relationship problems because the overloaded Heart chakra person is constantly giving but also constantly clinging, which ultimately pushes a more self-confident person away. Resentment and anger often build in a person with an overloaded fourth chakra because they aren't getting what they want, but they never express this for fear the other person will leave and they cannot imagine a life without the relationship. So they stuff the resentment deep down inside themselves, which leads to bigger problems down the line, such as depression. Often, these people get into *codependent* relationships with those who like this unequal balance of power, so that both people feed into each other's weak spots. For instance, an overloaded Power chakra person may be happy to take from an overloaded Heart chakra person, but that's not good for either one because it sends both out of balance.

def•i•ni•tion _____

Codependency is a term used in psychology to describe a situation in which someone becomes so preoccupied with giving to and caring for someone else that they neglect themselves. They believe that something or someone outside of themselves will make them fulfilled and happy. To these people, life is only okay if those around them are happy and well, thanks to their actions and care. Codependency is common in families of alcoholics, where the codependent person believes that if he or she works hard enough to help the alcoholic sober up, the family will be free of shame and anger. This only leads to disappointment because alcoholics sober up only when they decide to sober up, not because someone else worked hard to get them there.

Overloaded Heart chakras also tend to be overloaded in one direction only: outward. People in service positions, such as teaching, nursing, counseling, or the clergy, or those attracted to activist causes or charitable organizations, sometimes develop over-loaded Heart chakras because they spend so much of their energy focusing outward on the suffering of others. But when it comes to loving themselves, these people often are blocked. When all your heart energy pours out, you leave nothing left to nurture and heal yourself, and that results in a severe internal imbalance that will eventually deplete your energy and even impact the strength of your immune system.

Healing an Overloaded Heart Chakra

One great way to calm and balance an overloaded Heart chakra is to practice *prana-yama* breathing techniques. Especially, try this exercise called *Nadi Shodhana* for greater internal balance:

1. Sit comfortably and hold your right hand up. Curl your index and middle fingers in. Put your thumb next to your right nostril and your ring finger and little finger by your left nostril.

2. Gently close your left nostril by pressing your ring and little fingers against it as you inhale deeply through your right nostril.

3. After inhaling, pause as you release your left nostril and press your right nostril closed with your thumb. Exhale deeply through your left nostril.

4. Inhale deeply through your left nostril, then switch nostrils again, closing your left nostril and opening your right. Exhale deeply through your right nostril.

5. Repeat for two to five minutes.

Some other good strategies for healing an overloaded Heart chakra:

◆ Engage in self-care activities. Self-care is anything you do solely for yourself that brings you joy, happiness, and balance. Treat yourself to a massage, get a pedi-cure, take a walk outside in nature, sign up for that class you've been wanting to take. Do something *you* (not anyone else) want to do.

◆ Yoga poses that rein in your heart and relax and balance you can help. Try Child's pose (described in the "Child's pose (*Balasana*)" section), and Tree pose (see Chapter 7).

◆ Meditate for at least 5 minutes every day, working up to 15 or 20 minutes. Sit comfortably, relax, and practice watching your thoughts rather than letting them carry you away. With practice, you will begin to see that you are not your thoughts. They are only a small part of who you are. Let your mind relax and expand as you discover and explore your true beautiful nature.

♦ During meditation, use *mudras*. These powerful hand positions are designed to take the energy coming down your arm and re-route it back up so it stays inside your body and becomes more concentrated. Try *prana mudra:* Stretch out all your fingers, then bend your thumb and your ring and little finger so that the tips all touch. Leave your index and middle finger extended. Do this with both hands, and rest your hands, palms facing up, on your knees while sitting or on the ground while lying down. Breathe deeply.

def•i•ni•tion

Mudras are (most commonly) specific hand and finger positions that affect the internal energy of the body in specific ways. They are used in several ancient Eastern traditions, including yoga and Buddhism. **Prana mudra** is a *mudra* that joins the index and little finger tips with the thumb, to re-route *prana* back into the body for greater healing.

Yoga Poses to Balance the Heart Chakra

The best yoga poses for balancing both blocked and overloaded Heart chakras are those poses that help encourage balance. For blocked Heart chakras, work on backbends that open the chest. For overloaded Heart chakras, work on poses that draw heart energy within.

Bridge Pose (*Setu Bandha*)

Build a bridge to an open Heart chakra.

This pose opens the heart while maintaining safe, solid contact with the ground.

1. Lie on your back on the floor with your arms at your sides, your knees bent, and your feet on the floor. Move your heels as close to your body as you can while keeping your feet pointing straight out.

2. Inhale, and soften your body as you expand your heart center, literally relaxing your chest and letting it soften. Exhale and lift your hips up. Walk your shoulders side to side so that your shoulder blades can come more on your back body, and your chest and heart can begin to lift.

3. Clasp your hands underneath your hips and lift your hips a little higher as you focus on opening your chest. Try to keep your chin relaxed and slightly away from your chest. Keep your gaze looking up. Avoid turning your head side to side. Breathe deeply.

4. Hold the position for about 30 seconds, then slowly unclasp your hands and exhale as you come down.

Cobra Pose (*Bhujangasana*)

Open your heart from a position of strength.

This chest-opener is designed to mimic the shape of the cobra. As you do this pose, think about how an open heart doesn't have to mean a vulnerable heart. Opening your heart takes the strength and courage of the cobra.

1. Lie on your stomach with your palms on either side of your upper chest. Keep your legs together and press the tops of your thighs, shins, and feet into the floor.

2. Inhale and soften your body and mind. Exhale and push yourself up with your arms to raise your shoulders, head, and chest up off the floor. Curl into a baby back-bend. Flex the muscles in your arms as if you were going to drag

your hands back toward your hips. At the same time, push your chest forward. Imagine your Heart chakra's healing power flowing through your body. Hold for about 30 seconds.

3. Exhale and come down slowly, resting for about 30 seconds with your forehead on the floor.

Child's Pose (*Balasana*)

For a relaxing heart stretch, extend your arms in this variation of Child's pose.

This easy, nurturing pose is perfect for calming an overanxious heart and for restoring yourself when you are depleted from too much giving. Think of this pose as a great way to nurture your own inner child. Let this pose care for you in the same way you would care for any child in need of help.

1. Sit on your heels with your big toes touching, and widen your knees to the outside edge of your mat.

2. Exhale and bend forward to the floor. Bend your arms and fold your hands on the floor in front of you. Rest your forehead on your folded hands.

3. Relax in this position until you feel better.

The Least You Need to Know

◆ The condition of your fourth chakra represents your heart, your ability to give and receive love, your capacity to love yourself, and your sense of compassion and empathy for all beings.

◆ When the fourth chakra is blocked, symptoms include heart disease, lung problems, relationship problems, commitment issues, fear of intimacy, being judgmental, and an inability to feel compassion.

◆ When the fourth chakra is overloaded, symptoms include chest pain, breast problems including cancer, self-sacrificing behavior, codependency, and ignoring your own needs in the constant service of others.

◆ You can balance the fourth chakra by taking care of yourself, practicing breathing exercises, doing yoga poses that open the chest (like back-bends) or nurture the heart (like Child's pose), and by loving in better balance, giving and receiving love without sacrificing yourself or taking energy from your other chakras.

11

Throat Chakra (*Vishuddha*): Express Yourself

In This Chapter

- ◆ What your Throat chakra does, even without your help
- ◆ What your Throat chakra represents for your body, mind, and spirit
- ◆ How to tune in to your Throat chakra
- ◆ Correcting Throat chakra blocks and overloads
- ◆ Using yoga for Throat chakra fitness

Tell us *all about it*. Or can you? If you have an open and healthy Throat chakra, you can. The Throat chakra is the center for communication, sound, vibration, and ultimately, truth. This is where you express yourself in every way, and also how you receive the self-expression of others. People with strong Throat chakras have clear voices that people love to hear. This may also be expressed in a clear ability to write, draw, or express themselves with just the right words because people with strong Throat chakras tend to have good writing ability and musical ability. Many also have a good sense of rhythm and timing, not just musically speaking, but saying the right things at the right time. Our inner vibrations are expressed from this chakra, and so is our ability to be good listeners.

We all talk, listen, and understand others from this chakra. Through the Throat chakra, you understand not only what people say, but what they actually *mean*. You understand metaphorical and figurative language here. You also begin to understand the spirit.

The Throat chakra is the first of the spiritual chakras. Some people believe you can't open this chakra on your own, but instead need the guidance of a teacher. Others believe you can open your own Throat chakra with the right focus. This chakra is certainly different than the ones below it. Associations aren't as straightforward. This chakra, along with the two above it, enters the realm of the mind: vibration, visualization, intuition, and thought. What you say, what you see, what you imagine, and what you think are all reflected in the upper chakras, and it all starts here, with the fifth chakra, where your internal vibration is expressed through words, symbols, hand gestures, expressions—all the ways you communicate with the outside world. In this chapter, we look deeply into that place from which you speak to help you figure out what you know, what you understand, and what you *really* have to say.

Throat Chakra 101

The fifth chakra, also sometimes called the Throat chakra or Communication chakra, is called *Vishuddha* in the traditional Sanskrit. This word can be translated as "purity" or "purification." The traditional element associated with the fifth chakra is the ether, sometimes called space or the void—the place where nothing exists. Part of the understanding of the void in traditional yogic thought is that the void came out of pure sound vibration. The original sound that created the universe is the sound of *om*, and so some contemporary writers, such as chakra expert Anodea Judith, prefer to say that the element associated with the fifth chakra is simply sound.

def•i•ni•tion

Om, sometimes spelled *aum*, is a sacred symbol in Hinduism, representing the impersonal, omnipotent, absolute source of all creation. According to Hindu thought, the sound of *om* encompasses the past, present, and future and was the original vibration that created the universe. It is often used as a mantra in meditation or prayer, and speaking this intonation is thought to penetrate the soul.

The fifth chakra's symbolic color is blue and the traditional lotus symbol depicting this chakra has 16 petals. The sound associated with this chakra is the seed sound *HANG*. Chanting this sound helps to activate the fifth chakra.

The Throat chakra (Vishuddha).

The Throat chakra is located in the throat and encompasses the entire neck and upper chest, radiating around your jaw, mouth, ears, and down through your collarbones. Other physical structures associated with the fifth chakra are your thyroid, trachea, esophagus, parathyroid, neck vertebrae, and pharyngeal nerve plexus.

Let's Talk

What is talking? It's a strange ability we humans have. We make vibrations in our throats that come out of our mouths to make sounds that we all understand to symbolize other things. When you talk about a flower, the flower doesn't have to be anywhere near you. In fact, it doesn't even have to exist. But others who hear you (and speak your language) understand exactly what you mean. Language, including both speaking and writing, is all about symbols, and in the Throat chakra we begin to grasp the concept that one thing represents something else.

We understand this kind of symbolism in no simpler way than through what we say. Can you imagine how difficult it would be to function in the world today without being able to speak? If you've ever had laryngitis (a classic fifth-chakra issue), you know how frustrating it can be. Even the shyest among us need to speak. How else will anyone know what we need, what we want, *who we are?*

Your voice comes from your Throat chakra, and the quality of your voice says a lot about the state of your fifth chakra. A week, timid, shaky, or cracking voice indicates a blocked chakra, while a loud, booming, overpowering voice indicates an overloaded chakra. The condition of your voice isn't your fault, but it is a reflection of what is going on in your fifth chakra, which is, in turn, a reflection of what's going on within *you*.

When your fifth chakra is strong and healthy, your voice will be clear, pure, resonant, and pleasing to hear. People will enjoy listening to you speak and they will be likely to understand what you say (unless they have their own fifth chakra issues with listening). The fifth chakra reflects your ability to communicate your thoughts and intentions clearly and—just as important—to listen to and understand the expressed thoughts and intentions of others.

Energy Unplugged

When you were younger, were you allowed to speak your mind or were you told to be quiet all the time? Were children supposed to be "seen and not heard" in your home? Or was your home filled with too much talking, noise, yelling, and voices used to express negative emotions like anger? How you were raised to use or not use your voice is significant for the health of your fifth chakra today. Children who are discouraged not just from talking but from telling the truth, or who are told lies, often have fifth chakra issues as adults. Think about how talking, listening, and telling the truth were handled in your childhood home, to get a better feel for the state of your own fifth chakra.

Listen Up

Do you really know how to listen, or do you just wait to talk? Many people, when asked to consider the question, admit that they usually wait to talk. It's not surprising, really. In such a loud, raucous world, it's hard to get a word in edgewise and it can be easier to focus on getting your own words out than on letting others get theirs out.

However, knowing how to listen is a very important trait. If you balance the words you send out with the words you take in, you will feel calmer, more centered, and have a better understanding of your environment. Plus, listening is an important part of being a good friend, family member, and partner. It's also an excellent way to hone your intuition, which supports the health of your sixth chakra, the chakra governing intuition (see Chapter 12). Listening is powerful, and all you have to do to listen is stop talking and pay attention. It's worth a try.

Truth or Consequences?

You could call the fifth chakra the Truth chakra because this is also the place from where you speak your own truth, and discern the truth in what others say and do. This is a powerful skill, and one everybody possesses. Most of us don't use it like we could, though. When people constantly suppress their own truth—they don't say what they really mean or refuse to acknowledge something about themselves, for example—they often develop a block in the fifth chakra. To keep this chakra open and strong, spend the time to discover what really is true for you. Then spend the time to listen to what others say, including the meaning behind the words, and the meaning between the words, and soon you'll be hearing the truth, too.

Energy Unplugged

One way to hear the truth behind people's words is to pay attention not only to what they say but also to how they say it. People who study nonverbal communication say that nonverbal cues tell us more than the actual words people say. One study estimated that up to 93 percent of communication is nonverbal. To begin your study of nonverbal communication, start observing facial expressions, posture, what people do with their hands and feet when they talk, how they stand or sit, which way they lean, and what they look at. For example, people tend to lean toward things that interest them, and lean away from things they fear or don't like. They tend to blink a lot and not look people directly in the eyes when they are fudging the truth, and they tend to move more when they are nervous, less when they are engaged. See what you notice as you watch what people do, and whether it does or doesn't match what they say. Also pay attention to what your eyes, hands, feet, and body do when *you* talk.

Your Inner Music

The fifth chakra is about vibration and rhythm as much as it is about words. People with healthy fifth chakras often have nice singing voices (although not all of them do), and can carry a tune and keep a beat. Although their singing voice may not make them the next American Idol, people with open fifth chakras tend to enjoy singing, even if just in the confines of their own car! People with strong fifth chakras may have strong, unusual, sonorous, or memorable voices, not necessarily society's version of a *good* voice, but more of a *distinctive or interesting* voice. People who are tone deaf or who can't seem to hear rhythm or keep a beat very well may have blocked fifth chakras.

The entire universe is made out of vibration, and music is one of the most beautiful and poignant ways that we shape and celebrate vibration. Music is an excellent fifth chakra therapy, for both blocked and overloaded chakras, so listen to or play some music every day. It's good medicine for your fifth chakra.

Spinning Your Wheels

Betsy was working with a client who was a singer. She mentioned in therapy that she was having a difficult time with her voice. Sometimes her voice lost its strength, or became too nasal and shrill, and she couldn't seem to control when this happened. The woman also said that she found it very difficult to express the right emotion for the song she was singing, an essential part of being a good singer. Through therapy, Betsy discovered that this woman grew up in an abusive family where she was either ignored or told to "shut up and be quiet." She was literally prevented from having a voice as a child, and when she did try to express her feelings or emotions, she was punished for it. Thus, she learned to swallow her feelings because she had learned that expressing herself was bad. Yet, how interesting that this client chose a career path that forced her to use and develop her voice! Betsy says we often unconsciously choose the experiences we need most. As Betsy began to focus on the client's fifth chakra and free the energy here, the woman noticed almost immediate changes in her singing voice. Her tone became more even, and the strength of her voice became more powerful. Finally, she began to feel more comfortable exploring the emotions behind the songs she sang because her fifth chakra had opened.

The Write Stuff

Although the second chakra is an important source of creativity, so is the fifth chakra. Music comes from here, as does writing. Writers often have healthy, open fifth chakras because they constantly use them. A blocked fifth chakra can sometimes reveal itself through writer's block. In the same way that speaking uses spoken-word symbols to represent other things, writing uses written-word symbols. We all know how vivid and powerful a book can be, or even just a really descriptive paragraph. Words are our staircase to the mind, and writing helps you climb up there to look around. Writing, like music, is excellent therapy for both blocked and overloaded fifth chakras.

Energy Unplugged

If your fifth chakra needs work, or even if you just want to keep it healthy, try writing a little bit every day. Some people like to keep a journal of what they do and how they feel, while others would rather write stories, poetry, or an autobiography. What you write doesn't matter as much as just putting pen to paper or fingers to keyboard.

Throat Chakra Correspondences

Your voice, your words, your music, all of it ties together with the other fifth chakra correspondences. See them all at a glance in the following chart.

Fifth Chakra	
Sanskrit name	*Vishuddha* (purity)
Element	Space/the void, sound
Color	Blue
Seed sound	*HANG*
Location	In the throat
Associated cultural phrases	"Tell it like it is." "Speak of the devil and he will appear." "Speak up!" "Talk is cheap." "The sound of silence." "Silence is golden." "Truth or dare."
Associated anatomy	Throat, trachea, esophagus, neck, thyroid gland, pharyngeal nerve plexus, cervical spine, mouth, jaw, teeth
Associated psychological and life issues	Communication, ability to express feelings, ability to listen, speaking and hearing the truth, understanding meaning behind or beyond words, musical and writing ability
Physical issues related to fifth chakra blockage	Lump in the throat, laryngitis, sore throat, jaw pain and tightness, neck pain, stiff neck, neck arthritis, vocal nodes, recurrent strep, hypothyroidism, hearing loss, tinnitus, tone deafness (can't hear the difference between musical notes), no sense of rhythm

continues

continued

Fifth Chakra	
Psychological issues related to fifth chakra blockage	Problems with self-expression, weak voice, fear of speaking, lying, inability to discern the truth, inability to say what you mean, taking things too literally, writer's block
Physical issues related to fifth chakra overload	Hyperthyroidism; neck pain from hyperflexibility; vocal nodes from talking, yelling, or singing too much; tooth decay; tooth loss; cold sores; and canker sores
Psychological issues related to fifth chakra overload	Talking too much, talking too loudly, interrupting, speaking without thinking, inability to listen to others, automatically speaking the truth without sensitivity to others
Fifth chakra therapy	Mantra meditation, chanting, singing, drumming, speaking in front of others (for blocks), going without speaking (for overloads), quiet time, keeping a journal/freewriting, purposeful listening without commenting, practicing taking turns talking, lowering your voice (for overloads), raising your voice (for blocks), therapy for improving communication skills

Awakening the Throat Chakra

When your Throat chakra awakens, your voice becomes clearer, you say what you really mean, you listen to others and really hear them, and you discern the truth. Fire up your creative expression by literally opening your throat. Carefully tilt your head back and breathe. Feel your fifth chakra opening.

Another great, powerful way to awaken and energize the fifth chakra is through sound. Singing, chanting, humming, and saying mantras are all fifth chakra enhancers. Sing in the shower, hum while you make breakfast, and belt out your favorite tune in the car. Your fifth chakra will feel great.

To get more Throat chakra energy into your environment, emphasize the color blue. Wear bright sapphire-blue, paint your office blue, or put blue flowers around the house. Just seeing the color blue can help to awaken this chakra. Also include more sound elements in your home: wind chimes, noise machines that produce sounds such as waves or birds in a forest, and of course, music. Play music often to keep your fifth chakra energized.

You can also try this exercise for awakening the Throat chakra:

1. Sit on the floor, legs crossed, seat on a pillow or a folded blanket. Feel your pelvic bones and imagine roots anchoring those bones to the earth. Place your hands slightly behind you and move your shoulders back to open your chest.

2. Take several long, slow, deep breaths, and then draw your attention to the area inside your throat. Imagine your fifth chakra, a brilliant, sapphire-blue circle spinning slowly.

3. Imagine your chakra radiating a blue circle of brilliant light that encompasses your entire throat, jaw, and upper chest. Feel the cool electric blue in your throat, opening all your channels of communication.

4. Take a deep breath in and in a low resonating tone, say the word: *HANG*, holding the "A" sound (pronounced "ah;" the word rhymes with "song"). Repeat the word slowly sixteen times. Every time you speak the word, extend the sound as long as you can and feel the vibrations in your entire body, radiating from your Throat chakra.

Aligning the Throat Chakra

When your Throat chakra is properly aligned, you can use communication to help those you love, to improve your love relationships, and also to fully utilize your natural intuition. To get your Throat chakra properly aligned, try this exercise:

1. Stand in Mountain pose, with your feet about hip-width apart, arms at your sides.

2. Imagine your fifth chakra just behind your throat, and feel it spinning and getting cooler. Imagine a cool blue breeze blowing through your entire body.

3. Visualize a blue ray of light moving straight up out of your Throat chakra, up through the crown of your head, filling your head with blue light. Now, visualize this blue beam of light shooting straight down from your throat, down through your fourth, third, second, and first chakras and down into the earth. Imagine the entire ray of light filling your body with cool sapphire-blue energy.

4. Lift your arms straight up overhead and imagine the blue light flowing up and down, radiating to the center of the earth and all the way to the sky. Your chakra should now be aligned.

Blocks in the Throat Chakra

A blocked throat chakra can be a major impairment in our culture. It's the communication age, and those who can communicate effectively are usually well rewarded. People with blocked Throat chakras tend to be afraid to speak and have weak or quiet voices. They may come across as very shy. In our loud society, this can annoy people who might always be snapping, "Speak up!"

People with blocked Throat chakras also tend to have problems expressing their thoughts and feelings. People often misunderstand what they mean, and this can frustrate the blocked Throat chakra person so much that they are even more likely to clam up. Or they consistently say what they don't really mean. This is because they aren't willing to see and speak their own personal truth, or they fear a backlash or loss of love by speaking their truth so instead they say exactly what they think others want to hear.

Healing a blocked Throat chakra is incredibly important, not just to be able to communicate in society but to be able to express yourself. This is essential for psychological as well as physical health. Pent-up feelings and lack of acknowledgement of what is really going on can become major obstacles to contentment and well-being. However, some people fear what can happen if they really begin to speak. This fear can come from childhood experiences, or from a fear of consequences. And yet, the real consequences come from long-term stifling of truth and words. These clog up the body and can manifest as physical illness if you don't get them out. So let your Throat chakra open and set your voice, your words, and the truth free.

Blocked Chakra Health Issues

Fifth chakra health issues usually settle into the throat and neck. They can include such minor or temporary complaints as a lump in the throat, laryngitis, sore throat, strep throat, or a stiff neck, to more chronic problems like jaw pain and tightness, neck pain, arthritis in the neck vertebrae, stiff neck, neck muscle spasms, throat problems like vocal nodes or recurrent strep, and hypothyroidism. Your ears can also suffer from a blocked fifth chakra, which can manifest as tinnitus (ringing in the ears) or hearing loss, as well as being tone deaf, which means you can't hear the difference between musical notes, and having no sense of rhythm.

Blocked Chakra Psychological Issues

When the Throat chakra is blocked, the psychological implications usually have to do with self-expression. This can include speaking quietly or not using one's voice with conviction, fear of speaking in front of people, fear of speaking one's own truth, compulsive lying, inability to discern the truth in what others say, inability to say what one means, taking things too literally, and writer's block.

Sometimes you can spot someone with a blocked fifth chakra not only by the sound of the voice but by the way he tucks his chin in or bows his head, to protect the fifth chakra. You may even watch this type of person literally "swallow" her words. It's as if she wants to speak up, but the words get stuck and nothing comes out.

Energy Unplugged

When you lose your voice, consider that there might be something more going on than the common cold virus. People with blocked fifth chakras tend to be more vulnerable to colds, and their cold symptoms tend to settle in their throats. If you've lost your voice or have a sore throat, consider whether there is something you are not saying, or some truth you are refusing to see. Or maybe the problem is that you haven't been listening to someone, and your fifth chakra has literally intervened to make you stop talking so you can hear. Consider it a sign from your fifth chakra that something is awry in your communication system. (Of course, that doesn't mean you shouldn't drink a warm cup of tea and spend the day in bed!)

Healing a Blocked Fifth Chakra

To learn how to heal and strengthen a blocked Throat chakra, we turned to one of Betsy's colleagues, Joseph Mizelle, a licensed massage therapist, certified yoga teacher, and Reiki master and teacher who practices sound energy healing. Joseph has a beautiful voice and can make all kinds of amazing sounds, but his advice for people who need to unblock their fifth chakras is simple: sing. "Singing, humming, any kind of toning is activating and empowering for the fifth chakra," Joseph says. "This chakra is about creative expression, and just making sound gives people the opportunity to get in touch with what they need to say in their lives."

Don't worry if you think you can't carry a tune or you don't like your voice. Learning how to use it is key to unblocking your fifth chakra and freeing up your communication energy.

Joseph also suggests meditating on the fifth chakra and asking the body: "What am I not saying that I need to be saying?"

Then, start singing and see what comes out. You might be surprised at how relevant it is.

You can also try some of these activities to open a blocked Throat chakra:

- Call a trusted friend to get together and just talk. Be sure to listen, too.

- Eat blue foods like blueberries, blue corn chips, blue popcorn, and blue potatoes. (Naturally blue foods, not dyed foods!)

- Write someone a letter. You don't even have to send it. Just writing it will help open this chakra.

- Play music. Just turn on the radio, or play your favorite CD. Close your eyes and soak up the sound.

- Play a drum. Or just drum on a tabletop.

- Get a shoulder and neck massage.

- Recite these mantras: *I say what I mean. I speak the truth. Everyone hears me. I hear others. I express myself openly and freely.*

Energy Unplugged

Joseph Mizelle, sound energy healer, says that when you randomly start singing a song, the song that comes to mind is indicative of your psyche. In other words, the songs you choose to sing for no apparent reason often hold messages for you. Whenever you get a song stuck in your head or you latch on to a particular song you hear and start singing all day, stop for a minute and think about the words. What might they mean for you right now? Are they telling you what you aren't saying by yourself? Are they expressing your current mood? Are they solving a problem you have? In many cases, the answer to one of these questions will be yes. That's the power of sound, and your fifth chakra at work.

Overload in the Throat Chakra

If your problem is that you talk too much, too loudly, or you say things that aren't very considerate, you may have a Throat chakra overload. People with an overloaded Throat chakra have an entirely different kind of communication problem. They just can't stop talking.

These people talk over others, interrupt, dominate conversations, and are definitely more likely to be waiting to talk rather than listening. These people also use their voices in ways that hurt others. They may say too much, be unable to keep secrets, gossip, or even lie. We've all had times when we say more than we should have, but people with overloaded chakras do this chronically, and have a very hard time controlling the problem.

Overloaded Chakra Health Issues

An overloaded fifth chakra means there is too much energy in the throat. Physical signs of this can include hyperthyroidism (an overproduction of thyroid hormone), neck pain from being too flexible and wearing away cartilage between the vertebrae, and vocal nodes from talking, yelling, or singing too much. People who have to talk a lot in their professions can be prone to these problems, including professional singers, coaches, public speakers, and teachers.

Overloaded fifth chakras can also cause problems in the mouth, including tooth decay, tooth loss, cold sores, and canker sores.

Overloaded Chakra Psychological Issues

When you have too much energy in your fifth chakra, you will tend to talk too much, too loudly, and interrupt. People with overloaded fifth chakras speak without thinking first. Because of this, their words often hurt others. Just because something is true doesn't mean you have to *say* it. These people also tend to talk over others and aren't able to stop talking long enough to listen.

The problem with an overloaded fifth chakra is the way in which it compromises relationships, personal power, emotions, and even safety. In other words, an overloaded fifth chakra puts the health of all the lower chakras at risk. When you talk without thinking or say everything you are thinking out loud, people begin to withdraw from you. It's great to be able to express yourself, but you don't have to express every single detail of yourself. What about everyone else? Would you want to hear them talk about what is coming out of your mouth? Would you really be interested? Sometimes, silence is golden.

As for the upper chakras, how can you focus on your inner voice if your outer voice never stops talking?

In the same way that overloaded fifth chakra people need to back off a little bit and learn how to listen to others, they also need to learn how to listen to their own inner voice, which is quieter, but may have much more important things to say.

> **!!!** **Wake-Up Call** _____
>
> Eve has always been a talker, so it's no surprise she grew up to be a writer. She's had her fair share of chakra blocks, but her fifth chakra always seems to be wide open—maybe too open. When Eve was a child and her family went on car trips, they used to play the game, "Who can stay quiet the longest?" While Eve thought this was a fun and exceptionally challenging game, she had no idea that her parents were just trying to get a few blessed moments of silence! Eve now has her own kids, and her youngest son is the same way. He loves to sit and talk, and talk, and talk … and that's great! He's very good at self-expression. However, Eve now finds herself proposing that same game on car trips ….

Healing an Overloaded Throat Chakra

Healing an overloaded Throat chakra means burning off some of that excess vibrational energy, but unlike the lower, more physical chakras, the solution isn't exercise (except that if you are breathing hard enough, you probably can't talk!). Instead, the solution is simple: silence.

Take a vow of silence, even for just one hour. Or why not try a whole day of silence? Of course, some people can't be silent all day if they need to speak for their jobs or they have children. However, on a day when it could work, try it. Refusing to speak can be a transformative experience. You'll begin to hear things you never knew existed. You can keep a pad of paper and a pen handy for emergencies, but try not to use them. Unplug the phone. No text messaging or instant messaging or even e-mail— that's cheating. Stop the words and see what else lives out there in the world.

Some other good strategies for healing an overloaded Throat chakra:

- Meditate on the sound of your breath, or just sit quietly and listen to the sounds of the room without making any noise yourself. See if you can go for five minutes. Try to do this every day.

- Practice waiting three seconds to respond to any question or comment someone makes. This three-second wait time can allow you a space to breathe and consider what is appropriate and kind to say, rather than whatever random thing comes into your head first.

◆ Do people sometimes tell you to lower your voice? Try telling yourself first. Start to become aware of the volume of your voice relative to others. Can you dial it back?

◆ Practice listening like it's a sport. Spend some time every day consciously listening to someone who is talking to you. Make sure you understand what they are really saying before you respond. Try repeating back what they said, like this: "So, what I understand you to be saying is …." Rather than focusing your mental efforts on what *you* think of what they said, focus instead on what you think *they* think. (Got that?)

Yoga Poses to Balance the Throat Chakra

The best yoga poses for balancing both blocked and overloaded Throat chakras are those poses that physically open the throat. Even an overloaded Throat chakra can get into better balance through throat-opening poses, because these poses tone and strengthen the throat chakra, so it can better keep its normal shape. Think of it like a muscle that is either too tight or overstretched. Both can benefit from strength training.

Camel Pose (*Ustrasana*)

Moving into Camel pose opens the Throat chakra.

This pose opens both the chest and the throat, so it is perfect for fourth and fifth chakra balancing.

1. Kneel on the floor with your knees about hip-width apart. If this hurts your knees, kneel on a folded blanket. Focus on keeping your tailbone pointing straight down. Rest your hands on your hips.

2. Inhale and soften your body and mind. Exhale and release any fear or tension. On your next inhale, feel your side body or the space between your waist and armpit grow long, as your shoulder blades engage and come more onto your back body. Your heart lifts in an expression of openness and gratitude. Move your upper inner thighs back; you will feel your buttocks begin to stick out slightly. From here, scoop your tailbone down toward the mat, and feel your belly tone.

3. Keeping your hips in line with your knees, exhale and start to curve back. Your heart and chest begin to shine up toward the sky. Release your hands, stretch your arms down, and hold your heels. If you cannot reach your heels, rest your hands on your calves, or keep your hands on your hips, keeping the action of bending back and lifting the chest up.

4. Take your head back, if that's comfortable, and breathe evenly. Stay here for 10 seconds to 1 minute, depending on what feels best to your body.

To come out, lead with your heart. Place your hands back on your hips, inhale and lift from the heart, your head coming up last. After you are done, rest in Child's pose (see Chapter 10) for up to one minute.

Jhalandara Bandha

Tone the Throat chakra with this yoga bandha. *Bandhas* are interior body locks used in yoga practice, to help lock in and control the flow of *prana* or life force energy in the body. *Jhalandara bandha*, in particular, is perfect for toning the Throat chakra. Here's how to do it:

1. Sit in a cross-legged position on the floor. Relax.

2. Inhale so your lungs are about ¾ full. Hold your breath, then drop your chin down and draw it back toward your throat. This locks the breath in.

3. Hold this position (and your breath) for a few seconds, or as long as feels comfortable.

4. Raise your chin back to a normal position and exhale. Repeat a few times, working up to 16 repetitions.

The Least You Need to Know

♦ The condition of your fifth chakra represents your ability to communicate, express yourself, listen, speak truth, hear the truth, and understand the meaning behind and beyond words.

♦ When the fifth chakra is blocked, symptoms include a weak voice, laryngitis, throat pain, neck pain, stiff neck, jaw pain, hypothyroidism, dental problems, writer's block, lack of musical ability, and problems expressing yourself.

♦ When the fifth chakra is overloaded, symptoms include neck problems, hyperthyroidism, talking too much, talking too loudly, interrupting, and speaking without regard for other people's feelings.

♦ You can balance the fifth chakra by singing, humming, listening to music, writing, talking to people, listening to people, practicing silence, getting a shoulder and neck massage, and doing yoga poses that tone your throat.

Third Eye Chakra (*Ajna*): In Sight

In This Chapter

- What your Third Eye chakra does, even without your help
- What your Third Eye chakra represents for your body, mind, and spirit
- How to tune in to your Third Eye chakra
- Correcting Third Eye chakra blocks and overloads
- Using yoga for Third Eye chakra fitness

You know that *feeling* you get when the phone rings and you just know who it is? Have you ever been singing a song, and when you turn on the radio, that song is playing? Do you sometimes know what someone is thinking, or have a feeling something is about to happen, and then it does? Have you ever dreamed about someone, and then they contact you?

Life is full of these so-called coincidences, and according to yogic tradition, this "second sight" comes from the Third Eye chakra. Our two physical eyes see the past and the present. Our Third Eye sees the future. It's no coincidence that our "sixth sense" lives inside our sixth chakra.

The Third Eye chakra is the center, not just of our sense of what's coming, but of our intuition: what we *know* without seeing directly. As with the fifth chakra, we are now in the realm of the mind, rather than the body. The sixth chakra is the chakra of perception, imagination, and visualization, as well as dreams, visions, inspiration, and that inner voice we recognize as our conscience, telling us what is right and what is wrong. In India, people often mark the sixth chakra with a bright scarlet or yellow dot to help activate this chakra, but you can activate yours just by reading this chapter.

Third Eye Chakra 101

The sixth chakra, also sometimes called the Intuition chakra or Psychic chakra, is called *Ajna* in the traditional Sanskrit. This word can be translated as "command," although some people also translate the word to mean "perceive." The notion of commanding relates to the notion that the Third Eye contains not only our intuitive perception but our conscience—our perception is not necessarily neutral but has a sense of right and wrong and can guide us in how to act.

The traditional element associated with the sixth chakra is called *mahat*, which means supreme or great element. This is where all the elements combine into one. However, chakra expert Anodea Judith writes that this chakra is associated with the element of light. This makes intuitive sense because we cannot see without light, and we cannot "see" with our Third Eye chakra (in other words, tap into our own inner vision, intuition, and imagination) without an inner light to illuminate those perceptions. If the Third Eye chakra is closed, the light—our life force energy—cannot penetrate through and we are in inner darkness.

The sixth chakra's symbolic color is sometimes described as a deep indigo, and sometimes described as purple. Throughout this chapter, as you tune in to your own sixth chakra, use your intuition to discover which color rings more true to you. The traditional lotus symbol depicting this chakra has just two petals, on either side of a central circle, like two eyes on either side of the Third Eye. The sound associated with this chakra is the seed sound *AUM*, the original, primordial sound of universal vibration. Chanting this sound helps to activate the sixth chakra, as well as to bring unity to all the chakras.

The Third Eye chakra is located just between or slightly above the eyebrows and encompasses the entire face and head. Other physical structures associated with the sixth chakra are your pituitary gland, pineal gland, carotid nerve plexus, brain, eyes, nose, and sinuses.

The Third Eye chakra (Ajna).

I See ...

What do you see? Just the objects around you, or do you see more? Although you could list things you see in front of you, you might have trouble putting into words everything you "see" as you move through your life. You see a sunrise, but you also "see" that your friend is worried about something. You see a math problem, but then you suddenly "see" how to solve it. You see someone you love in front of you who is trying to explain how they feel. Then you "see" what they mean.

The Third Eye chakra is all about what you see, in every sense of the word. It influences your physical eyes and your imagination, your ability to perceive information both literally and metaphorically, and your inner wisdom that sees what has to be done. It's all going on right there in the middle of your forehead.

Psychic Moments: Your Intuition

What is being psychic? Many believe those who are psychic simply have a more finely honed intuition. Intuition is the part of you that picks up on cues in the environment that are so subtle, your conscious mind doesn't even notice them. You "get a feeling" you should cross the street, or avoid that lane of traffic, or get out of the elevator when someone else gets in, or call your mom.

Energy Unplugged _____

Children have amazing imaginations, but they also have amazing perceptions. They see things adults don't always perceive with their busy, stressed, crowded brains. Sometimes children may misinterpret the things they see, but if they are constantly told that what they see doesn't exist, they quickly learn to stifle their perceptions and ignore their intuitions. When a child thinks she sees a ghost, or believes his dream really happened, or tells you that grandma was in his room when grandma lives in another state, or is quite sure she knows exactly what her goldfish is trying to tell her, imagine what happens when a trusted parent says "You are wrong." If you were told that your childhood visions weren't real, you may have learned not to listen to your inner voice or heed your inner vision. Children whose visions are acknowledged, considered, discussed, and honored, even if the adult ends up explaining what might really be going on, learn that their own Third Eye might really know something after all. That's an empowering gift to give a child.

Some of what you might be picking up are mental pictures that come through your sixth chakra. When the sixth chakra is open and healthy, your intuition can speak up and encourage you to take notice. Don't ignore it. Studies show that people who follow their intuition are more likely to avoid dangerous situations. Those who ignore the sixth sense because they think they are just being silly or paranoid or overly sensitive often find out too late that their intuition was spot on.

Imagination Station

Remember all the things you used to imagine as a child? Imagination is fun, but adults often push it to the side or forget about it entirely. Yet our imaginations—even if they lie dormant—stay with us for our entire lives and people with healthy, open sixth chakras have an all-access pass.

Adults can use their imaginations in many productive and wonderful ways, from daydreaming and pass-the-time fantasies to actually charting a course for the future, whether that has to do with career development, relationship improvement, retirement planning, or how to finally live your dream, whatever it is. People in creative professions use their imaginations regularly, but it doesn't have to be limited to the realm of your job. If you let your imagination work for you, it will. This is the place inside yourself where you can do and be anything. Using your imagination can be just plain fun, without the aim of manifesting the things you imagine. However, if you want to live your dreams, if you want to make what happens in your head happen in your life, begin here. If you imagine it, then you might just be able to make it so.

Picture This

If you've ever taken a yoga or meditation class, you have probably experienced *visualization*. Your mind's ability to see what isn't actually there is reflected in the state of your sixth chakra. From here, you can form mental pictures of anything from the things you want the most to the things that most frighten you.

def•i•ni•tion

Visualization is the act of forming mental images of something, for various purposes. Some people use visualization to help with centering, relaxation, or focus during meditation. They might visualize a calming environment such as a beach, a meadow full of flowers, or a mountaintop with a beautiful view. Some people use visualization to help something actually happen in their lives, such as visualizing money coming to them or visualizing being at their ideal weight. Elite athletes have been known to visualize consistently making the free throw or making the perfect putt. Some people use visualization to enhance creativity, or they do it just because it's fun.

Some people find visualization easy, particularly those with healthy sixth chakras. For others, picturing something that isn't there is challenging, but energizing the sixth chakra can help. Practice helps, too. The more you use your imagination to visualize the things you want to see, the more skilled at visualization you will become. It's enjoyable to picture things in your mind, from memories of happy times in the past to visions of places you would like to go and things you hope to achieve someday. Visualization can even help you find solutions to your problems and ways to overcome obstacles in your life. It's a powerful tool, and all you need to do to start learning is to close your eyes. (Or you could check out *The Complete Idiot's Guide to Creative Visualization* by Shari L. Just, Ph.D., and Carolyn Flynn.)

Many of the exercises in this book require visualization. Every time we ask you to visualize one of your chakras as a certain color, or spinning, or radiating, or anything else, that's visualization.

If this has been difficult for you (or even if it hasn't), try this powerful exercise. It's excellent for honing your visualization skills, and can also help you use your intuition to discover some new things about yourself:

1. Sit comfortably and close your eyes. Take a few deep breaths.

2. In your mind, picture yourself descending a long staircase. At the bottom, you come to a hallway with three doors on each side of the hallway and a door at the end. All the doors are closed.

3. Imagine walking down the hallway, looking at each door. Every door looks a little different. Try to imagine the details of each door.

4. Now, choose a door and open it. Let yourself imagine what you see behind that door. Walk inside the space you imagine and take as long as you like to visualize every detail. Is it an ornate living room? A meadow full of flowers? A room of glass and steel? A balcony overlooking the mountains? Or something completely abstract? Whatever it is, let yourself examine your surroundings for as long as you like, adding details as you go. Use all five of your senses to help your visualization take form. What smells are behind the door? Are there certain sounds unique to this place? What colors do you see? Do you have a taste in your mouth connected to this place? What does your body feel like, physically, when you are here? Your inner vision may not be complete at first, but that's okay. When you've spent as much time as you want to spend in the room of your imagination, go back out the door into the hallway, and open another door. Step in and visualize this new place.

5. Continue with this visualization until you have opened every door in that hallway. Visualize the space behind each door as well as you can. After you are finished, sit for a few minutes thinking about what you saw behind each door in your mind, and what it might mean in your life right now.

Wise Up

As much as the sixth chakra is about seeing, in all its many manifestations, it is also about knowing. This is where wisdom lives, as well as conscience. Through your sixth chakra, you not only see what is going on, but you know what it means. You understand if it is right or wrong, and you also simply understand it. You are wise in your sixth chakra. Close yourself off here, and you lose not only your moral compass, but also your ability to make a decision based on more than just surface-level knowledge. An open sixth chakra allows you to tune in to your ah-ha moments of recognition, discovery, and understanding. Here, you can tap into a deep inner and eternal knowing. Close it off and you lose this center of wisdom.

Spinning Your Wheels

Carol generally had an open sixth chakra, but over the course of about a month, during regular sessions with Betsy, Carol's sixth chakra was consistently closed. Upon exploration of this, Carol admitted that a past lover had resurfaced in her life. Several months earlier, she had experienced a brief, yet serious and intense, relationship with him until she learned he had a serious girlfriend in another state. Since the old lover had made contact again, Carol found herself fantasizing that they could live happily ever after, and that he would eventually leave his girlfriend (even though he still had not done so). In therapy, Carol was able to finally see how her sixth chakra had closed down because she didn't want to hear her inner wisdom that this man was not good for her.

Dream On

Sometimes, what we see in our dreams can seem just as vivid as what we see when we are awake. Dream energy lives in the sixth chakra, and tuning into your dreams is an excellent way to energize the Third Eye. Each morning, try to remember your dreams, and think about what they might tell you, to get a new perspective on what is going on in your life. Dreams speak in symbols and pictures, and what they tell you is wise. (For even more help on interpreting your dreams, check out *The Complete Idiot's Guide Dream Dictionary*, which Eve co-authored with Gayle Williamson.)

Energy Unplugged

Anyone can develop better dream recall. Keep a journal and pen next to your bed, so that you can write down visual impressions from your dreams the moment you wake up in the morning. Before you go to sleep, tell yourself you will remember your dreams.

Third Eye Chakra Correspondences

Tap into your inner wisdom by becoming aware of the many areas of your life that correspond to your sixth chakra.

Sixth Chakra	
Sanskrit name	*Ajna* (purity)
Element	All elements combined, light

continues

continued

Sixth Chakra	
Color	Indigo or purple
Seed sound	*AUM (OM)*
Location	Between and just above the eyebrows
Associated cultural phrases	"Sixth sense." "What you see is what you get." "Picture this." "I see what you mean." "Seeing is believing." "She has second sight." "Use your head." "Get out of your head." "Don't lose your head." "You are living in a dream world." "His head is in the clouds." "Get your head screwed on straight."
Associated anatomy	The brain, nerves, forehead, eyes, nose, pituitary and pineal glands, and the carotid nerve plexus
Associated psychological and life issues	Intuition, perception, wisdom, imagination, ability to visualize, dreams
Physical issues related to sixth chakra blockage	Headaches (including migraines), nasal congestion, sinus infections, near-sightedness and other problems seeing clearly, night blindness, stroke due to blockage, brain tumor, head injury (can cause a blockage)
Psychological issues related to sixth chakra blockage	Lack of imagination, can't remember dreams, no intuition, chronic bad decision-making, denial of reality/self-deception, sociopathic behavior.

Physical issues related to sixth chakra overload	Headaches (particularly from dilated blood vessels), hallucinations and other visual disturbances involving seeing things that aren't there, hyperventilation, brain hemorrhage, brain tumor, head injury (can cause an overload)
Psychological issues related to sixth chakra overload	Psychic visions that interfere with normal life, can't tell dreams from real life, disconnected from reality, psychosis, being "too much in your head"
Sixth chakra therapy	Visualization, meditation, drawing and painting, practicing tuning in to your intuition, keeping track of your dreams, therapy to help clarify your inner vision, *hypnosis*

def•i•ni•tion

Hypnosis is a state of altered consciousness during which there is increased focus and a greater openness to suggestion. Although people can hypnotize themselves (self-hypnosis), typically another person such as a therapist guides the person into the hypnotic state. Hypnosis can be used to treat many physical and emotional conditions such as anxiety, migraine headaches, phobias, and chronic or acute pain. Hypnosis can also help people tap into their intuition. Look for a mental health practitioner who specializes in hypnosis if you want to explore this powerful way to get in touch with your sixth chakra.

Awakening the Third Eye Chakra

When your Third Eye chakra awakens, you become more perceptive and intuitive. You notice more of those little signs that urge you in the right direction, and your inner voice becomes clearer. People with awakened Third Eye chakras also tend to have exceptionally creative imaginations, good vision, and can remember and understand their dreams.

Awakening your Third Eye chakra can be as simple as touching your forehead to the ground, but meditating, drawing or painting, keeping track of your dreams, or practicing visualization are all great ways to get the Third Eye chakra activated.

To get more Third Eye chakra energy into your environment, highlight the color indigo, or deep purple. Wear indigo, paint the room where you meditate indigo, or put deep purple flowers around the house. Also include more light elements in your home: interesting light fixtures, candles, or crystals and prisms that hang in the window and catch the light, throwing rainbows on the wall.

You can also try this exercise for awakening the Third Eye chakra:

1. Kneel on the floor; bring your big toes together and your knees wide apart. Put a folded blanket in front of you.

2. Bend forward and rest your forehead on the blanket. Close your eyes. Take several long, slow, deep breaths, and then draw your attention to the area inside your Third Eye. Imagine your sixth chakra, a brilliant, deep indigo-purple color, spinning slowly. See if you can feel a vibration on your forehead, where it touches the blanket.

3. Take a deep breath in and in a low resonating tone, say the word *AUM* slowly, two times (pronounce this in three parts, holding each part for a few seconds, like: *ah-oh-oomm*). Feel the word vibrating into your sixth chakra.

4. Rest quietly with your head down for a few minutes, imagining the deep indigo color spinning in your forehead.

Aligning the Third Eye Chakra

When your Third Eye chakra is properly aligned, your intuition will become fine-tuned. You'll be able to hear your inner voice and heed its wisdom. To get your Third Eye chakra properly aligned, try this exercise:

1. Stand in Mountain pose, with your feet about hip-width apart, arms at your sides.

2. Imagine your sixth chakra in your forehead, between and just above your eyebrows. Visualize a deep indigo curtain opening to reveal your radiating sixth chakra.

3. Visualize a deep indigo ray of light moving straight up out of your Third Eye chakra, up through the crown of your head, filling your head with indigo light. Now, visualize this indigo beam of light shooting straight down from your Third Eye, down through your fifth, fourth, third, second, and first chakras and down into the earth. Imagine the entire ray of light filling your body with indigo energy.

4. Lift your arms straight up overhead and imagine the light flowing up and down, radiating to the center of the earth and all the way to the sky. Your chakra should now be aligned.

Blocks in the Third Eye Chakra

When your Third Eye chakra is blocked, you just don't *notice things*. Not only is your intuition blocked, so is your direct perception. Have you ever looked for something, like your car keys, and then suddenly you see them right in front of you on the table, even though you swear you already looked there? Has someone ever tried to send you subtle hints and had to resort to kicking you in the shins because you just didn't pick up on what they were trying to tell you nonverbally? Do they say you can't take a hint? Have you ever been startled because somebody snuck up on you, even though in reality, you just didn't see or hear them approaching? These are all signs of sixth chakra blockages. It's that feeling that you are "checked out" or just don't have your head screwed on straight.

Blocked Chakra Health Issues

Sixth chakra health issues usually settle into the head. Headaches (including migraines), nasal congestion, sinus infections—anything that physically blocks up the processes in your head can be related to sixth-chakra blocks. So are visual problems, such as a sudden onset of near-sightedness, night blindness, blurred vision, and other problems seeing clearly. Brain abnormalities can be reflected in a blocked sixth chakra. A head injury can also precipitate a blocked sixth chakra.

Blocked Chakra Psychological Issues

When the Third Eye chakra is blocked, the psychological implications usually have to do with a lack of perception and imagination. People with blocked Third Eye chakras seem to have no "vision"—for their own futures, for the world, or even for what they want to accomplish at any given time. Or they may seem practical but not creative because their imaginations are stifled. Visualization is difficult for people with sixth chakra blocks, and they rarely recall their dreams.

These people are often in denial. They don't want to see what is going on in their lives, perhaps because they believe it is too painful, so they close themselves off to their inner vision and their inner voice. They might ignore their conscience, or continue on in a bad situation because it is easier or more comfortable than seeing the truth. They don't seem to realize that listening to and following their own intuition, which resides in the sixth chakra, will lead them to their best possible life.

> **Energy Unplugged**
>
> To help unblock your sixth chakra, keep a drawing journal. Use a journal with unlined pages or a sketchpad and a pencil. Take 10 or 15 minutes to draw anything that comes into your mind. The point is to focus on the visual and translate what you see to paper. Even if you think you can't draw, give it a try

People with a blocked sixth chakra also tend to proceed through life as if they have blinders on. They seem to be narrow-minded because they only see things one way or perceive things to be black and white, with no shades of gray. They have trouble perceiving subtle differences in things or accepting that there are exceptions to every rule. They miss out on much of the complexity and diversity of life because seeing it is too difficult or painful, or they never really learned how to see the world through that Third Eye lens.

Healing a Blocked Sixth Chakra

To heal and strengthen a blocked Third Eye chakra, focus on honing your vision, both outer and inner. Really look at things. Tune in to the colors and shapes in your environment. Close your eyes and visualize places, people, and situations. Try to visualize things that could never actually happen or places you've never actually seen. Fantasize. (How often is someone going to tell you to do that for your health?)

You can also try some of these activities to open a blocked Third Eye chakra:

◆ Paint. Watercolors and acrylics are easy to use. Experiment with color. Don't worry about skill, just have fun seeing.

◆ Keep a dream journal and write down dream impressions each morning. The more regularly you try to remember your dreams and write down the images you recall, the more you are likely to remember.

- Eat dark blue and purple foods like purple and black grapes, eggplant, plums, red cabbage, and blackberries.

- Try wearing a blindfold for a while. See how your perceptions change without your outer vision.

- Have someone give you a head rub, or get a facial massage.

- Spend time in a steam room breathing deeply.

- Recite these mantras: *I can see clearly. I have an inner vision. I trust my inner voice. I listen to the deep and eternal wisdom that resides within me.*

Energy Unplugged

Beauty may be in the eye of the beholder, but that shouldn't stop you from celebrating whatever *you* think is beautiful. Looking at beautiful things is incredibly therapeutic and excellent for unblocking the sixth chakra because it makes seeing highly rewarding. We're not talking about being obsessed with superficial beauty. We're talking about things that radiate inner beauty. Gaze at a beautiful view, take a walk in a beautiful setting, stare at a beautiful sky, whether it's bright blue or dark and speckled with stars. Look at and appreciate beautiful objects, beautiful animals, and people you think are beautiful, or who are doing something beautiful, like dancing, skating, or just sitting and thinking.

Overload in the Third Eye Chakra

For some people, the Third Eye chakra takes over and visions are all they have. A sixth chakra overload can be a real problem for someone who has to function in the world. Overloaded Third Eye chakras can reflect hallucinations, delusions, and obsession with memories of the past. If you live in a fantasy world, spend too much time daydreaming, or have a lot of trouble focusing on your current situation and environment, you may be overloaded in your sixth chakra.

People with overloaded Third Eye chakras sometimes have psychic abilities, or think they do. However, these inner visions impair normal life because the person experiencing them can't distinguish them from outer visions. These people may also have such vivid dreams that they mistake them for reality, or they may have terrifying nightmares that stay with them, and which they can't stop replaying in their minds. These are the people who are so convinced their visions are true that they skew their own intuition, taking every leap of imagination as "a sign," and every visual image as a dire warning or prediction.

Overloaded Chakra Health Issues

People with overloaded sixth chakras tend to have headaches caused by dilated blood vessels, such as tension headaches. They may suffer from hallucinations and other visual disturbances that involve seeing things that aren't there, including extremely vivid dreams. In extreme cases, they may experience a brain hemorrhage or other brain abnormalities. As with sixth chakra blocks, a head injury can also cause a sixth chakra overload.

Overloaded Chakra Psychological Issues

When you have too much energy in your sixth chakra, you tend to be so focused on your inner vision that you can lose touch with the real world. In extreme cases, a sixth chakra overload can indicate *psychosis*, signaled by a total break from reality. More commonly, however, the overloaded Third Eye chakra person tends to be overly tuned in to intuition and the inner voice, to the point that this focus interferes with normal life. Sixth chakra overloaded people also tend to think too much, at the expense of acting. If this is you, people might sometimes tell you to "get out of your head" or "stop thinking so much."

def·i·ni·tion

Psychosis is a mental disorder characterized by failure to recognize what is real and what is not real, to the extent that the psychotic person cannot function in everyday life.

If you have an overloaded sixth chakra, you may also have extremely vivid dreams and usually remember many of them in the morning. Keeping a dream journal can be helpful for you, too, not to help you remember more but to help you process all those images. Write down what you remember, and think about what it might mean for your real life. Are your dreams solving problems for you, urging you to get out and act on them?

Healing an Overloaded Third Eye Chakra

First-chakra grounding can be helpful for an overloaded sixth chakra. Get into your body more and you'll have an easier time balancing your tendency to live inside your head. Exercise, preferably outside where you can focus on beautiful surroundings. Take a walk through the woods or a park. Tune in to what is really there, rather than spending the entire time thinking about other things.

Consciously working to be present is excellent for an overloaded Third Eye chakra. Pay attention to where you are, what you are doing, and what is going on around you periodically throughout the day. When you focus on your physical environment and the task at hand instead of always living in your head, thinking about the past or the future, you will not only help to heal your Third Eye chakra but you will also notice that you can concentrate better and get things done more efficiently. An overloaded Third Eye chakra can definitely predispose some people to chronic multitasking. Your mantra: *one thing at a time.*

Some other good strategies for healing an overloaded Third Eye chakra:

♦ Practice *mindfulness meditation*, a form of meditation in which you sit and observe your present state from moment to moment, without letting your thoughts carry you away to some other mental place.

♦ Practice noticing what physically exists around you. Remind yourself periodically throughout the day to "be here now." Take a "vision break" every two hours and spend just two minutes observing actual objects in your immediate environment.

♦ Go back and review Chapter 7, which is all about the first chakra. The stronger your first chakra, the better you will be able to remain grounded, and the less you will be stuck in your head or ruled by the sixth chakra. These two chakras balance each other in many ways.

Yoga Poses to Balance the Third Eye Chakra

The best yoga poses for blocked Third Eye chakras are those poses that encourage *pratyahara*, the yoga principle of withdrawing the senses and turning inward. The yoga poses that help to balance an overloaded Third Eye chakra are those that encourage grounding in one's physical surroundings. Following, we've included a few of each.

def•i•ni•tion

Pratyahara is the yogic principle of withdrawing the senses from external objects to focus on the inner vision. This is one of the Eight Limbs of Yoga, as described by Patanjali in the *Yoga Sutras*. Regular sensory withdrawal results in greater control over the senses, so they are not mistaken for more than they are.

Sensory Withdrawal Poses

We've already introduced you to two great poses that are perfect for withdrawing the senses to focus on the Third Eye chakra. One is Child's pose (see Chapter 10). Rest your forehead on the floor or on a folded blanket during this pose, and focus your attention on the Third Eye.

The other pose is Corpse pose, described in Chapter 7. In this pose, as you lie perfectly still and relax every part of your body, focus on the Third Eye chakra and try to feel it. Let this chakra become your point of focus, so that all your senses converge here, energizing and awakening your inner vision.

Grounding Poses

The poses best for balancing an overloaded sixth chakra and bringing the mind back into the body are those that require maintaining concentration and balance. Any balancing pose, such as Tree pose (Chapter 7), works to help shrink the sixth chakra down to size.

The Least You Need to Know

- The condition of your sixth chakra represents your ability to see, use your intuition, use your imagination, remember your dreams, listen to your inner voice, and heed your conscience.

- When the sixth chakra is blocked, symptoms include vision problems, headache, nasal congestion, sinus infection, stroke, brain abnormalities, lack of imagination, difficulty with visualization, rarely remembering your dreams, lack of intuition, and no sense of inner voice or conscience.

- When the sixth chakra is overloaded, symptoms include headache, hyperventilation, brain hemorrhage, hallucinations, psychic abilities that impair normal functioning, psychosis, living in a fantasy world, being "in your head" too much, and problems distinguishing dream experiences from real experiences.

- You can balance the sixth chakra by drawing, painting, meditating, visualizing, recording and interpreting your dreams, paying attention to what you see around you, listening to your intuition, and doing yoga poses that withdraw the senses (for blocks) or are grounding (for overloads).

Crown Chakra (*Sahasrara*): Thousand-Petaled Lotus

In This Chapter

◆ What your Crown chakra does, even without your help

◆ What your Crown chakra represents for your body, mind, and spirit

◆ How to tune in to your Crown chakra

◆ Correcting Crown chakra blocks and overloads

◆ Using yoga for Crown chakra fitness

To be a whole person with complete body-mind-spirit integration, one must involve the seventh chakra—the part that reflects the human spirit. Spirit means a lot of different things to different people, and in the context of the seventh chakra, it also has a range of meanings.

This is the realm of higher brain function, so not only does the seventh chakra reflect our connection (in a traditional sense) with the higher power or universal energy that some people call God, but it also reflects our "big picture" sensibility. The impulse to understand who we are and where we fit into the broad scheme of things comes out of the seventh chakra. This place where we question the meaning of life, as well as the place where we learn tegrate what we learn into who we are. This is also where we receive inspira-, sudden a-ha moments of understanding, and a deep sense of connectedness to all life and the energy that connects all life. We may not feel it all the time, but when we get those flashes of unified feeling, they come from the Crown chakra.

Betsy rarely sees people with closed seventh chakras, and she believes this is because we are all deeply connected to each other and to universal energy, even if we don't realize it consciously.

Crown Chakra 101

The seventh chakra, also sometimes called the Crown chakra, Spiritual chakra, or Thousand-Petaled Lotus chakra, is called *Sahasrara* in the traditional Sanskrit. This word is usually translated as "thousand-petaled" or "thousand-spoked," referring to the thousand petals of the lotus flower that symbolically represents this chakra.

Traditionally, this thousand-petaled lotus is pictured not as sitting upright atop the head but as inverted on the crown of the head, with the thousand petals extending downward. The lotus is an ancient symbol for spiritual flowering because it floats in ponds and its roots extend deep down into the mud at the bottom of the pond. In the same way the lotus is rooted in murky mud but produces a beautiful white flower above the surface of the water, so must we be rooted in the sometimes dark and murky physical world, but have the potential to blossom spiritually.

However, the fact that the lotus flower is inverted on the body in its traditional representation also suggests that this chakra is rooted in heaven and extends down to each of us, as if the divine presence, spirit, or God has reached down to touch you reassuringly on the crown of the head. This is your connection to something greater than yourself, and your sacred proof that you are an integral part of that greater something.

There is no traditional element associated with the seventh chakra, which extends beyond the physical notion of earthly elements, although chakra expert Anodea Judith says the element of this chakra is thought itself. Just as we touch spirit here, we also expand the mind, which is the tool that enables us to understand and communicate with God or universal energy.

The seventh chakra's symbolic color is sometimes described as purple, and sometimes described as pure white. As you work with your own seventh chakra, use whatever color makes sense to you. The traditional lotus symbol for this chakra is typically depicted sitting inverted on the crown of the head. There is no element associated with the Crown chakra, there is also no literal sound. Instead, the seed sound of this chakra is the sound of God or the universe speaking *AUM*, rather than a human voice saying anything at all. Some people also interpret the seed sound of the seventh chakra to be the sound of breath. It is typical in chakra meditations *not* to speak when reaching this chakra. Instead, feel the universal vibration speaking it.

The crown chakra (Sahasrara).

The Crown chakra is located slightly above the crown of the head. It encompasses the brain and especially the cerebral cortex, the external layer of gray matter that covers the cerebrum and cerebellum. The cerebral cortex is the most highly developed part of the brain, responsible for the most advanced of human brain functions like thinking, understanding, and integrating information.

Will the Real You Please Stand Up?

Who are you? This is probably a question you have thought about periodically throughout the course of reading this book, but the question is never more relevant than when you are working with your seventh chakra; this is where all the parts of you come together. In some systems of belief, spirituality is something separate from the physical, and physical reality is considered unreal or inferior or, even worse, something to deny. However, the concept of the chakras defies this ideology. From the first through the seventh, each chakra represents an integral part of who you are, and each part develops out of the one below it, so that by the time *Kundalini* energy reaches the Crown chakra, you can experience complete integration of all your parts: your instincts, your physical urges, your feelings, your relationships, your compassion, your communication with others, your intuition, and your place in the universe.

Within your seventh chakra, you have the capacity to see all these parts together and integrate them into one exciting, fascinating, and endlessly revealing *you*. Even as you connect to something greater, that doesn't obliterate who you are. Rather, it enhances and clarifies you.

Energy Unplugged

Spirituality is easy for kids. Spiritual visions and perceptions seem unsurprising to them. However, a child's spirituality is a delicate and sacred thing. Children who grow up in a restrictive religious environment often have later difficulty with spirituality, especially if they reject their childhood religious experience and retain negative memories from it. Conversely, children with absolutely no spiritual experience may have a hard time opening up to spirituality later in life because it is foreign territory that never had a chance to develop. While every parent has different priorities, the most important way to help a child's seventh chakra develop in a healthy way is to never deny them the reality of their own spiritual perceptions.

The Spirit Link

The nature of the spirit is complex and takes our highest brain function to understand. Even then, we can probably only hope to scratch the surface of what it means. Different cultures define spirit in different ways, too—as something within, or something outside of us, or both.

The Crown chakra encompasses our connection both to our own spirituality and to a universal spirit that exists within and beyond us. The seventh chakra is like a door that opens to welcome God, or universal life force energy. Call it what you want to call it, envision it in whatever way works for you, but the sense is the same. We are a part of something bigger, and we join with this greater energy through our seventh chakras. We send who we are out this door, and the universe sends what we are back in, so that we recognize we are part of something. We are never alone because of this sacred link.

For those who don't spend much energy on spiritual pursuits or who were never raised in a religious tradition, this can be a difficult concept to swallow. Don't worry about that. If the seventh chakra doesn't speak to you—if you don't feel like you need it right now—that's fine. It is still open, giving and receiving like a great cosmic modem, linking you to everything else that has ever lived, breathed, existed. Trust in that, if you want to. Or don't worry about it until you need to. For some, understanding the Crown chakra may come through the lens of your religion, but the Crown chakra does not have to be related to religion. Whatever way you look at it, it is about connection.

The Religion Connection

Betsy has worked with many clients on issues relating to religion. She believes that religion can be an incredibly positive force, and although it isn't for everyone, for some people it is healing and supportive. Sometimes, however, people can develop anxiety and other issues connected with negative religious experiences. In these cases, the Crown chakra can provide a lifeline.

Betsy had a client named Sarah who was having panic attacks. Saddled with frequent anxiety, the college student came to see Betsy because her anxiety was interfering with her life. Through therapy, Betsy learned that Sarah was raised in an extremely religious household that emphasized sin and an angry, punishing God. Sarah always had huge fears of letting down God and being subject to his wrath. She had vivid memories as a child of being told that if her behavior didn't change, she would go to hell. She regularly experienced fear, guilt, and shame, related to the way religion was practiced in her childhood home.

As she matured, Sarah began to feel so oppressed by the moral expectations placed upon her by her church and her parents that she began to separate from her childhood church and from her family. Eventually, Sarah abandoned anything to do with religion and spirituality and decided the only way she could progress was to become an atheist (someone who does not believe in God).

As Betsy began to help Sarah explore her belief systems, it became obvious that Sarah was in mourning. She was grieving the loss of the idea that there was some higher power in the universe and that she was connected to this powerful force. Sarah was missing the positive aspects of religion because she had rejected the entire concept, rather than just those parts that had hurt her in the past. Instead of fearing sin, Sarah's anxiety stemmed from her fear of isolation from God.

Sarah had decided that the God of her childhood no longer fit into her worldview, so she thought that meant there could be no God. However, Betsy discovered that from the very first session, Sarah's seventh chakra was open and strong. Sarah found this difficult to believe. How could her spiritual chakra be open when she was an atheist who had purposefully cut herself off from anything spiritual?

As they worked, Sarah began to re-evaluate the meaning of her open and balanced seventh chakra. Week after week, as her chakra remained open, she began to feel a sense of relief that maybe she was still connected to a higher power after all.

During therapy, Betsy helped Sarah to clarify what she was really feeling, and to discover that it was not necessary for her to carry the same strict religious beliefs her parents held in order to have a spiritual life. As an adult, she could figure out what spirituality and God meant to her.

Sarah began to practice meditation to connect with a larger life force. With regular meditation practice, Sarah rediscovered her spiritual self and was able to free it from the chains of negativity based in her past. Her anxiety eased and she felt more calm, balanced, and integrated.

Higher Education

The seventh chakra also governs your ability to learn. All knowledge you take into yourself comes in through the Crown chakra, which also reflects the state of the cerebral cortex. You know what they say: never stop learning. To energize this chakra, keep learning. When learning stops, this chakra falters. Fortunately, for most people living an active and interactive life, learning never stops because knowledge isn't just about taking a Spanish class or learning to play the guitar or going back to get your degree. It is about engaging with the world and discovering what that means for who you are and what you are becoming at any given moment.

The Big Picture

When you are conscious, your seventh chakra is at work. In this way, the seventh chakra encompasses a wide range of thought, from philosophical musing to simply being awake. When you are unconscious, such as while you are sleeping, if you faint, or if you are in a coma, your seventh chakra closes. But you don't necessarily have to be asleep to be walking through this world in an unconscious state. Wake up to your life and live with intention and engagement, and it opens again.

Seat of the Soul

Not everyone buys into the idea that each of us has a soul, something apart from our physical body that survives after our bodies die. For those with open seventh chakras, however, the presence of the soul is self-evident. You can just feel it. For those who have been around someone who has died, you may even have seen or sensed the soul leaving the body as that person took the last breath (not always at the exact moment of physical death, sometimes just before or just after).

Spinning Your Wheels

In 1907, Dr. Duncan McDougall, a Massachusetts physician, theorized that the soul was an actual thing with weight, and famously measured bodies just before and just after death. The doctor carefully accounted for moisture loss and other factors, but discovered that at the moment of death, some of the bodies he measured suddenly dropped in weight by about three-quarters of an ounce, more or less. While the six people he measured make for a pretty small sample group and his experiments had many flaws, the notion that the soul weighs 21 grams (the amount the first body he measured lost at the moment of death) comes from Dr. McDougall's experiments.

While nobody has ever proven the existence of the soul, many people believe that the soul is the part of you that lives within your body but is not part of your body. You can't see it on an x-ray or even measure it with a pendulum. It is the presence of life force energy within you, imprinted with your individual signature, but also with the signature of the universe, like a contract jointly signed.

In other words, the seventh chakra reflects not only the body's consciousness, but the spirit's consciousness, too. The Crown chakra is the soul's home, and the state of the soul—not whether it is "saved" or "damned," which are concepts foreign to yogic philosophy, but what it says about spiritual health—is reflected in the energy of this chakra.

Crown Chakra Correspondences

Your spiritual life is reflected all over your physical life, and the Crown chakra has many correspondences that can help you tap into its power. These correspondences are summarized in the following chart.

Seventh Chakra	
Sanskrit name	*Sahasrara* (Thousand-Petaled)
Element	No element; or, thought
Color	Purple or white

continues

continued

Seventh Chakra	
Seed sound	The divine speaks the sound; or, the sound of breath
Location	At the crown of the head
Associated cultural phrases	"That's the spirit!" "Believe in me." "You've got to have faith." "God willing." "Look at the big picture." "I think, therefore I am."
Associated anatomy	The skull, brain, cerebral cortex
Associated psychological and life issues	The true self, unity in all things, knowledge and understanding, spirituality, connecting to a higher power or universal energy, seeing the big picture, the soul
Physical issues related to seventh chakra blockage	Learning disabilities, nervous system failure, headaches (at the crown of the skull), autism, brain tumor, coma, amnesia, senility/Alzheimer's disease
Psychological issues related to seventh chakra blockage	Feelings of isolation, depression, lack of inspiration, spiritual crisis/"dark night of the soul"
Physical issues related to seventh chakra overload	Headaches (at the crown of the skull), Savant Syndrome, brain tumor, overactive nervous system, seizures, health problems related to poor hygiene or physical neglect

Psychological issues related to seventh chakra overload	Obsession with or addiction to spiritual or intellectual practices, religious/spiritual delusions/hallucinations, nervous breakdown, uncontrolled out-of-body experiences, dissociation with the body, over-intellectualizing, feeling ungrounded
Seventh chakra therapy	For blocks: meditation, prayer, spiritual study, self-study, learning something new and challenging like a musical instrument or a language, therapy to deal with spiritual crisis. For excess: grounding, balancing all seven chakras, physical exercise, therapy to reintegrate the mind with the body, therapy to put spiritual beliefs and practices into perspective.

Awakening the Crown Chakra

When your Crown chakra awakens, you see beyond the limits of your own ego. The universe gets bigger and begs the question: "Why?" The lifelong quest to answer that "why" is the province of the seventh chakra; your Crown chakra is the tool for uncovering the answer. Learning, experiencing new things, seeing things in a new way, and generally expanding the mind more and more to encompass each new facet of life as it is encountered, are all activities that awaken the Crown chakra. Ultimately when the inner gaze turns even more fully outward and beyond human experience to seek meaning in a broader, universal perspective, the question becomes: "Who is running this show?" or "What drives it all?" or "What is the nature of the fuel for this energy?" or, simply, "What is God?"

You nudge your Crown chakra open every time you gain new knowledge or experience. Whenever you reach out into the universe with a question, your seventh chakra comes to life.

To get even more Crown chakra energy into your environment, highlight the colors purple or white. Wear these colors, use them in your home, and fill your home with the tools for gaining knowledge, like books and computers. Also consider reserving a space in your home for meditation or prayer, where you can be quiet and reflect on things. A meditation room is nice, but not necessary. Any space that is clean, uncluttered, and quiet will work. Use it every day and your Crown chakra will remain open and strong, a conduit for universal energy.

You can also try this exercise for awakening the Crown chakra:

1. Kneel on the floor and put your palms together in front of your chest, in prayer position.

2. Bow your head in supplication to an energy greater than yourself. Close your eyes. Take several long, slow, deep breaths, and then draw your attention to the area at the crown of your head.

3. Raise your head up so your neck is in line with your spine. Imagine your seventh chakra. Try to see what color it is, deep purple or bright white. Imagine it glowing brilliantly and spinning slowly. Try to feel it at the top of your head, or just above it, as vibrating energy.

4. Breathe evenly and listen to the sound of your breath. Now, imagine God, or universal vibration, uttering the sound: *AUM*. Don't make any sound yourself, other than breath. Just listen and hear the sound coming from outside yourself but vibrating inside you.

5. Once again, bow to divine energy, then rest your hands on your knees, lift your head, and open your eyes.

Aligning the Crown Chakra

When your Crown chakra is properly aligned, you feel both grounded, connected to others, and connected to the universe. You perceive the unity in all things, and yet appreciate your own individuality and ability to gain knowledge and interpret information as part of your personal growth. Aligning your Crown chakra is the final act of alignment; when all your chakras are straight, open, and permitting the free flow of life force energy, you will gain ultimate balance. You can live in the world, but also know God.

To get your Crown chakra properly aligned, try this exercise:

1. Stand in Mountain pose, with your feet about hip-width apart, arms at your sides. Feel your feet firmly planted on the floor. Connect with the energy of the earth, imagining yourself becoming grounded.

2. Imagine your seventh chakra at the crown of your head. Visualize a deep purple or pure white light shining out of the top of your head, extending in a brilliant beam up toward the sky. Imagine energy flowing up out of your seventh chakra, and then imagine a matching beam of light coming down from the sky, from far beyond the place where you could see the source, and beaming right into the crown of your head so that energy is flowing up and down.

3. Now, visualize this beam of light shooting straight down from your crown, down through your third eye, your throat, your heart, your solar plexus, your navel, and out from the base of your spine, straight down into the earth. Imagine the entire ray of light filling your body with glittering, radiating energy.

4. Lift your arms straight up overhead and imagine the light flowing up and down, into heaven and down from heaven, into the center of the earth and back up again. Your seventh chakra—and all your chakras—should now be aligned.

Blocks in the Crown Chakra

When your Crown chakra is blocked, you feel cut off. It's as if someone cut the power to your house and your source of energy and heat is gone. With a blocked Crown chakra, you can still function in the world. You can talk to other people—even love them. You can feel and do and speak. However, you cannot speak to God, you cannot feel a connection with the life force, and you will have trouble seeing the big picture, even learning. You won't have any context for your knowledge. Your spirit is stifled and you feel lost, even when you know exactly where you are.

Fortunately, Crown chakra blocks aren't common. The universe has a way of whispering to us even if we aren't listening. Even if we give up on God, or that universal life force, it does not give up on us. It takes powerful negative experiences to close a Crown chakra, but when it closes, you may experience a spiritual crisis. The question "What does it all mean" suddenly seems like it has no answer, and the consequences of that nonanswer may suddenly seem more dire than you ever imagined.

People with blocked Crown chakras also tend to have problems learning. They have trouble grasping new concepts and settle into such a comfortable sameness that the idea of experiencing anything new becomes terrifying. Healing a blocked Crown chakra is incredibly important, not just to be able to live fully but to be spiritually whole. Your whole brain can't function properly without an open Crown chakra.

Blocked Chakra Health Issues

Seventh chakra health issues, like sixth chakra health issues, settle in the head, but have more to do with the top of the head and higher brain function. A blocked Crown chakra can result in headaches, especially those on the top of the head. The sudden onset of learning disabilities, memory loss (like amnesia), or other brain dysfunction are common with seventh chakra blocks. So is any temporary loss of consciousness, including coma.

Blocked Chakra Psychological Issues

When the Crown chakra is blocked, the psychological implications relate to both learning and spiritual matters. Blocked seventh chakra people have trouble comprehending new information and sometimes isolate themselves in order to avoid dealing with the repercussions of a learning disability or cognitive malfunction. They may refuse to see beyond a narrow set of beliefs or to experience anything new. Even some religious people have closed seventh chakras because they actually worship their own narrow idea of God rather than being open to the experience of actual divinity. This can happen out of fear, force of habit, or simply a lack of courage and curiosity. The result is often narrow-mindedness, prejudice, hate, depression, and a life that gets smaller and smaller.

Blocked seventh chakras are also related to spiritual crisis, common when someone rejects a spiritual tradition and has nothing to take its place, or becomes filled with doubt and experiences the classic "dark night of the soul," in which all previous faith is called into question. When someone gives up on learning, rejects new knowledge, or turns away from the spirit, the seventh chakra can shut down.

Mother Teresa's much publicized spiritual crisis is a perfect example. Her words to the Reverend Michael Van Der Peet in September 1979 express this block: "Jesus has a very special love for you. As for me, the silence and the emptiness is so great that I look and do not see, listen and do not hear." Even though she was famous all over the world for her selfless work and spiritual life, even she had doubts, fear, and a feeling of isolation from God.

Energy Unplugged _____

You don't have to be religious to have an open seventh chakra. You don't even have to believe in any particular God, or even the concept of a higher power. Many people are spiritually connected to life force energy despite their rejection of organized religion or what they think of as spiritual pursuits. Some are so devoted to *not* believing in God, or to logic or science or secular humanism, that this devotion becomes, in itself, a sort of religion of the mind and generates its own brand of spirituality. Even being passionate about living, learning, and being is a reflection of an open seventh chakra. In other words, the seventh chakra does not demand any particular adherence other than the one devoted to the quest for knowledge of the meaning of life. When the quest for knowledge is active, so is the seventh chakra.

Healing a Blocked Seventh Chakra

To heal and strengthen a blocked Crown chakra, work your mind by gaining knowledge. Purposefully have new experiences, even if you don't necessarily find that comfortable. Think, consider, philosophize, theorize, and never stop learning. Let your quest for knowledge encompass both the physical world and the world beyond. Question what you learn and don't just believe everything you hear. Be open to not only facts but also those realities that may not be provable. Have both doubt and faith, and a willingness to see beyond the obvious. If it's good for your brain, it's good for your seventh chakra.

You can also try some of these activities to open a blocked Crown chakra:

♦ Meditate, especially on the nature of the universe, God, or any other spiritual matters you find interesting. Try listening for the answers to your deepest questions.

♦ Pray or reach out to a higher power in whatever manner fits in with your belief system. Ask for what you need and want. The Universe will hear you.

♦ Learn something new. Studies show that learning a language or a new musical instrument are two of the best ways to maintain cognitive brain function.

♦ Eat purple or (naturally) white foods like purple grapes, plums, purple or white eggplant, white radishes, potatoes, or onions.

♦ Catch snowflakes or raindrops on your tongue, or take off your hat and feel them landing on your head.

♦ Do word or number puzzles.

- Have someone give you a head rub.

- Recite these mantras: *I can learn anything. I honor my body, my mind, and my spirit equally. I am filled with life force energy. God lives within me. I am a divine being. I never stop learning.*

Overload in the Crown Chakra

When the Crown chakra is too open and overloaded with energy, spiritual matters not only prevail, they push other matters off the radar. These are the people who get addicted to religious practices or are so overzealous in their spiritual pursuits that they forget to live in the world. This is fine for monks and nuns in monasteries and hermits in caves who have devoted their lives to the singular pursuit of spirituality, but for the rest of us who have to live in the world, a sense of balance with the more mundane aspects of life is essential (for that matter, even monks and nuns need to make the food, do the dishes, and weed the garden). An overloaded seventh chakra tips the scale away from the real world, the body, and even other people, in favor of a vision that always and only looks upward.

But an overloaded Crown chakra can also be about an obsessive devotion to learning and gaining knowledge at the expense of actual practical application of knowledge. People with unusual intellectual abilities sometimes have overloaded seventh chakras when these abilities control their lives. Maybe you are so devoted to spiritual pur- suits that you don't remember to eat, sleep, or brush your teeth. Or maybe you are a scholar, an intellectual, or so fascinated with learning that you spend your days Googling questions on the Internet, reading political blogs, or plumbing the depths of sacred texts to find answers to your most philosophical questions. Whatever the case, an overloaded seventh chakra can result in being completely out of touch with the real world, your actual body, your job, your daily duties, and your relationships.

Overloaded Chakra Health Issues

People with overloaded seventh chakras tend to have headaches at the crown of the head, rather than in other areas like the forehead or sinuses. An overloaded seventh chakra sometimes can be reflected in a brain abnormality, especially one that grows quickly. Savant Syndrome, a condition characterized by having unusual skill at some- thing such as art, music, math, or remembering dates, can be a sign of an overloaded seventh chakra, if that person is (as is often the case) impaired in other ways. Howard

Hughes comes to mind—a brilliant thinker and doer, a genius, but yet saddled with obsessive-compulsive disorder and other problems that made it extremely difficult for him to live a normal life.

People with overloaded seventh chakras can also have overactive nervous systems and can suffer from seizures or nervous breakdowns. Because they often lose touch with their bodies, people with overloaded seventh chakras may also have poor hygiene or health problems related to physical neglect.

Overloaded Chakra Psychological Issues

When you have too much energy in your seventh chakra, you tend to be so focused on your mind that you lose touch with your body, which can cause not just health problems but problems with relationships and daily functioning. If you forget to shower or change your clothes, you are probably going to start having problems out there in the world.

Overloaded seventh chakra people also tend to be addicted to spiritual or intellectual practices like prayer, meditation, or constant study. They may suffer from religious or spiritual delusions or hallucinations, and may even have out-of-body experiences because they are so much in their heads and so little in their bodies. They may also feel separate from their bodies, as if their bodies don't belong to them. Over-intellectualizing is a common problem for overloaded seventh chakras, and so is a feeling of not being grounded.

> **!!! Wake-Up Call**
>
> If you have an overloaded seventh chakra, chances are you have a closed first chakra, because these two chakras often reflect each other's imbalances. Likewise, an overloaded first chakra sometimes coincides with a blocked seventh chakra. To balance your Crown chakra, look back at the exercises for energizing and opening your Root chakra.

Although we are all spiritual beings having a human experience here on earth, it is important to remember that we are also living on the physical plane within earthly bodies and we need to pay attention to the body and the world around us, rather than constantly focusing exclusively on the spiritual world beyond.

Healing an Overloaded Crown Chakra

First-chakra grounding can be very helpful for overloaded sixth and seventh chakras. Get into your body more and you'll have an easier time balancing your tendency to live inside your head. Move your body, feel your feet on the ground, jump up and down, dance, and exercise. Pay attention to the world. List physical details you see in front of you. Touch things. Smell, taste, feel. Remember, you are here in your body right now for a reason. You aren't up in heaven yet, or even in an ivory tower. Live while you are alive. It isn't all about thinking.

Some other good strategies for healing an overloaded Crown chakra:

- Practice balancing all seven chakras each day, to remind you that you are more than just your brain.

- Tune in to your five senses. Sit quietly and focus on everything you can see in the room around you. Then, notice everything you can hear, from the sound of traffic or birds outside to the creaking floors and ticking ceiling fan. Next, tune in to everything you can feel: the air on your face, your clothing, your jewelry. Can you smell anything? Breathe in deeply and find out. What taste do you have in your mouth right now?

- Eat something. Eating is very grounding. Foods that come from the earth, especially those that grow deep in the soil like potatoes, onions, and carrots, are especially grounding. Eat slowly and notice the taste and texture of the food.

- Exercise outside. Get your heart rate up and your muscles moving.

- Therapy can help you reintegrate your mind and body, or help you to put your spiritual or intellectual practices into perspective so you can also function in the real world.

- Practice noticing what physically exists around you. Remind yourself periodically throughout the day to "be here now." Take a "vision break" every two hours and spend just two minutes observing actual objects in your immediate environment.

Yoga Poses to Balance the Crown Chakra

Two good yoga poses for balancing the Crown chakra are Corpse pose (*Savasana*), which you first learned in Chapter 7, and Headstand pose, also called *Sirsasana*.

When doing Corpse pose to balance the Crown chakra, focus on the feel and weight of your body sinking into the ground, but also envision your crown opening and energy flowing through all your chakras.

Headstand is an advanced yoga pose and we don't encourage you to try it for the first time on your own. Go to a yoga class where an experienced teacher can lead you safely into this pose. However, go ahead and try our easier variation, explained in the following.

Modified Headstand (*Sirsasana*)

A full Headstand pose draws blood to the head and nourishes the Crown chakra.

If you've been practicing yoga for a while and a skilled teacher can demonstrate to you, in person, how to do headstand, then go for it. Headstand against a wall is a great place for people to start who are ready for this pose. Eventually, you may even be able to do a Headstand in the middle of the room. This is an excellent pose for both opening a blocked seventh chakra and calming an overloaded seventh chakra, because it puts your portal to the mind directly in contact with the earth.

However, not everybody can do Headstand pose, or can't do it yet. Why not get all the benefits without all the pressure? Try this modified version:

1. Kneel on all fours in front of a folded blanket. Place your hands on the blanket and come down onto your forearms. Clasp your hands together making a space about the size of your head with your hands. Keep your elbows wide apart and make sure your wrists stay pushing down into the blanket.

2. Raise your hips and come onto your feet so that your hips are in the air, your feet on the ground, and your upper body is supported by your forearms and hands.

3. Put your head down into the space between your forearms so your crown rests on the blanket and your clasped hands cup your head. Walk your feet in a little closer. If this is too difficult, come out of the pose and move to a wall, so your back can lean against the wall as you walk your feet in closer to your arms. Or don't come up onto your feet. Stay on your knees as you rest your head on the floor.

4. Take a few deep breaths and feel the crown of your head against the blanket. Stay in this position as long as you like.

5. To come out of the pose, come back down onto your knees with your forehead resting on the floor. Stay here for at least 30 seconds. Sit up slowly.

The Least You Need to Know

- The condition of your seventh chakra represents your intellectual ability, your spirituality, and your connection to spirit, God, universe, or a higher power.

- When the seventh chakra is blocked, symptoms include the sudden onset of learning disabilities, nervous system failures, headaches, brain abnormalities, coma, amnesia, feelings of isolation, depression, lack of inspiration, and spiritual crisis.

- When the seventh chakra is overloaded, symptoms include headaches, Savant Syndrome, brain abnormalities, overactive nervous system, seizures, nervous breakdown, health issues related to poor hygiene or physical neglect, addiction to spiritual or intellectual practices, religious delusions or hallucinations, out-of-body experiences, dissociation with the body, over-intellectualizing, and feeling ungrounded.

- You can unblock the seventh chakra by meditating, praying, spiritual study, learning new things, or therapy to help deal with spiritual crisis. You can balance an overloaded seventh chakra by doing grounding and first chakra energizing activities, physical exercises, tuning in to the five senses, eating, and therapy to reintegrate body and mind or to put spiritual practices into perspective.

Part 4

High Octane Bliss ... No Caffeine Necessary!

Once you really know your own chakras and what's going on inside, you can have some chakra fun. In this part, you learn about how to increase your energy through chakra work, use mantra, chanting, and other sound techniques to resonate through and further awaken your chakras, and even explore how your chakras relate to your sex life with some enlightening Tantric techniques. This part ends with a chapter on meditation, one of the best ways to get in daily touch with your own chakras and integrate them into your life.

Chapter 14

Energize: How Chakras Help You Feel Better

In This Chapter

- Chakras and energy
- Why chakra work feels good
- Using chakras for better sleep, pain relief, and anxiety management
- More courage and better concentration through chakra work
- Chakra weight loss plan

You can understand what chakras are, what they do, how they work, and what aspects of you are reflected in each one, but we know that what you really want to do is to be able to use them to make your life better. That's what this chapter is all about.

Energy on Tap

If you have read these chapters in order, you've already learned how energy moves through the meridians in your body, pooling and circulating in your seven primary chakras. This energy comes into your body with the breath, and the chakras transform that energy into something you and your body can use.

The way each chakra translates *prana* is unique. The first chakra turns energy into instinct, the will to survive, courage, a sense of security, and the ability to make yourself safe. The second chakra transforms energy into passion, creativity, and connection. The third chakra turns energy into personal power and action. The fourth chakra transforms energy into love, compassion, and the will to care for yourself and others. The fifth chakra makes energy into messages and channels creativity to the outside world. The sixth chakra turns energy inward to access inner wisdom and intuition. Finally, the seventh chakra sends energy out into the universe so you can find your place in the scheme of things.

When you have to deal with real-life challenges each day, the different ways your chakras transform energy can be immensely helpful because you have access to that energy. You can use this energy even more effectively when you customize the energy you need for the task at hand. You wouldn't put jet fuel into your car, eat gasoline for lunch, or heat your home with a sandwich. You also wouldn't plumb the depths of your first chakra to hone your intuition or tap into your seventh chakra for better digestion.

But chakra energy isn't exclusive to a single chakra, either. Many issues can best be served by tapping into the energy from more than one chakra, boosting the power of each in a way that makes the energy from several chakras greater than the sum of its parts.

Your chakras are energy centers that correspond to nerve centers in the body.

Feel-Good Power

Working with your chakras makes you feel good for a variety of reasons. First and most obvious, chakra work helps to open blocked chakras and ease the pressure on overloaded chakras, so energy flows unimpeded through your body. When every part of you gets its fair share of *prana*, you feel better than you do when part of you and part of your life gets too much or too little energy.

Chakra work also feels good because it requires you to pay attention to *you*. It's easy to put yourself at the bottom of your priority list, especially when you have to take care of other people and multiple responsibilities in your life. The more you increase your internal energy supplies, the more effectively you can provide for the people who depend on you.

Chakra work literally feels good, too, because when you have a physical problem, such as insomnia, chronic pain, anxiety, or fear, accessing energy from the right chakras can solve the problem, or support and facilitate your other efforts to work on your issues. Here are some ways to use chakra energy to make your life work better.

Getting Your Zzz's

Americans are chronically sleep-deprived. According to the National Sleep Foundation's 2008 Sleep in America poll, the average time Americans spend asleep is just 6 hours and 40 minutes per night, even though the recommended amount of sleep is 7 to 9 hours. Because this is an average, that means that a lot of people get even less sleep.

Too little sleep isn't always just a matter of having too much to do or watching TV too late at night. People with *insomnia* can't fall asleep or stay asleep, even when they try. Not only is this inability to fall asleep a miserable experience, but it also has been linked to physical illness, chronic pain, depression, and anxiety, among other issues.

Because insomnia can cause so many problems, from daytime sleepiness and lack of focus to anxiety, depression, and irritability, solving a sleeplessness problem can make a big difference in your life.

def•i•ni•tion

Insomnia is a sleep disorder characterized by problems falling asleep or staying asleep. Insomnia is almost always due to stress and tension in a person's life that prevents them from falling asleep. However, insomnia can also be caused by a sleep disorder such as sleep apnea. Thus, discussing your sleep problems with a physician is important so you can determine the cause of the difficulty getting those zzz's.

Sleep is a survival act. Our bodies require sleep for physical healing, emotional balance, and mental decluttering. That means the energy for sleeping comes primarily out of the first or Root chakra, the place that reflects your survival instinct. Fear and a deeply rooted sense of insecurity can also be reflected in the first chakra, and if these issues contribute to sleeplessness, then the healthy energy of the first chakra can help to resolve this barrier to a good night's sleep.

In addition to the first chakra, other chakras are related to insomnia because insomnia occurs when the mind can't stop chattering. Thinking is the realm of the sixth or Third Eye chakra, and anxiety happens here. This is also the chakra that energizes and influences our dreams, which helps to process mental activity. With insomnia, there is typically too much energy in the sixth chakra, and a lack of energy, or grounding, in the first chakra.

To receive the best, most regenerative sleep possible, get your energy moving down from your sixth chakra into your first chakra as a way to decrease some of the anxious energy in your mind.

Try this whenever you are having trouble getting to sleep. As with other exercises, you can record your own voice or someone else's reading these cues, or just read them over a few times so you can guide yourself silently.

1. Lie down on your bed, or any other place where you would like to fall asleep. Lie on your back and move your shoulder blades underneath you, as if they are cradling your heart. Let your arms rest at your sides, palms facing up, leaving about a foot of space between your hands and the sides of your body. Stretch your legs out, then relax them and let them fall open.

2. Breathe softly, feeling your breath flow in and out but not controlling it.

3. Bring your awareness to your feet. Notice everything about your feet. Are they warm or cold? Can you feel socks on your feet or are you barefoot and experiencing the weight of your sheet and blankets on your feet? Begin to experience your feet becoming heavy and warm, so heavy that your feet feel as if they are sinking into the surface upon which you rest.

4. Now visualize a warm red glow at the base of your spine. The light is comforting and makes you feel at home. It turns slowly, anchoring your body to the ground, and you experience its red glow descending down each leg into both of your feet, warming them. Imagine this light is protecting you, keeping you safe, and shielding you from any danger or insecurity.

5. When you feel secure in this red glow, move your attention to your forehead. Imagine a deep indigo glow like an evening sky filled with sparkling stars, slowly rotating like a galaxy over your forehead. Visualize all your scattered thoughts running around inside your head. Imagine the indigo light gently surrounding the scattered thoughts. All the chattering energy in your mind is quieted by this indigo light, and the excess energy here is transported down to your feet. Now imagine the indigo light forming a shield that extends beyond your body and beyond the red shield so that your entire body is encased in a two-layered cradle of red warmth and dark starry sky.

6. Now, imagine you are being gently rocked to the rhythm of the planet's spinning. Your first chakra still anchors you to Earth and provides safety, while your sixth chakra keeps thoughts far away from you, launching you safely into a sweet, quiet sleep filled with regenerating energy and gentle, nurturing dreams.

7. Staying relaxed, let yourself stay in this quiet place for as long as you need to stay. If you feel compelled to turn onto your side or stomach, that's okay, but if the new position starts to make you restless, return to your back. If you fall asleep, then congratulations! Your chakra energy provided your body with what it needed. If you didn't fall asleep, that's okay, too. This kind of deep relaxation is almost as regenerative as actual sleep.

Easing the Pain

Pain is also a first chakra issue because our bodies launch into survival mode when we feel pain. However, the fourth or Heart chakra is the healing chakra. Combining survival energy with healing energy can banish or at least help ease pain, no matter what the cause.

If you suffer from chronic pain, carefully read the chapters on chakras one and four, and work on the exercises provided in those chapters to energize, align, and balance those chakras. Accessing your inner resources for survival and healing can make a big difference if you work on these chakras regularly.

Sometimes, though, you might be suffering from a flare-up or temporary pain from an injury. Or maybe you have an emotional wound. Both physical and emotional pain can benefit from this quick healing exercise, so try it whenever pain is distracting you from what you are doing. It will only take two minutes.

You might find this exercise even more effective than aspirin.

1. Sit, stand, or lie down in a comfortable position that does not aggravate your pain. Relax as much as you can. Close your eyes.

2. Take a slow, deep inhalation through your nose, taking about 10 seconds to fill up your lungs. Pause for five seconds and imagine the energy from your held breath lighting your Root chakra like a struck match flaring into flame.

Wake-Up Call

If you have a medical problem or suffer from severe pain but aren't sure why, please consult a doctor, in addition to trying any chakra exercises.

3. Exhale slowly through your mouth, taking about 10 seconds to empty your lungs. As you exhale, imagine the spark spreading into a warm red glow all around your Root chakra, getting warmer and brighter, as if fueled by a bellows filled up with the air of your exhaling breath.

4. Keep that idea of warmth at the base of your spine, then inhale again for 10 seconds. Pause for five seconds and imagine that held breath igniting your Heart chakra like a struck match.

5. Exhale slowly, taking about 10 seconds to empty your lungs. As you exhale, imagine the spark in your Heart chakra spreading into a bright green flame that surrounds your heart.

6. Inhale one more time, slowly for a count of 10 seconds, and imagine the warm red glow rising and the warm green glow descending until they meet in your solar plexus, right in the middle of your Power chakra. Hold your breath for five seconds and imagine the energy from your first and fourth chakras combining and strengthening.

7. Exhale one more time, slowly for a count of 10 seconds, and imagine that healing power you've generated pouring into the part of your body that hurts. Allow each exhale to be a release of pain and discomfort. Feel the warmth as your body begins to heal itself and the pain begins to float far, far away. Visualize that energy knitting the broken pieces back together and putting everything back in line. Move your body in any way that it feels like it wants to move, such as shifting positions, sitting up straighter, or standing up. Your own healing energy may be making adjustments to your physical body.

8. Breathe normally for a few more breaths and continue to feel healing energy processing and eliminating your pain. When you are ready, open your eyes.

Calming Down

Sometimes stress gets the best of all of us and we find ourselves freaking out. Whether you are having a full-blown anxiety attack or just pacing back and forth, incapacitated by worry or excessive negative energy, your chakras can help process and eliminate some of that overload so you can feel calmer faster.

Anxiety often comes from your first chakra, if you feel scared or unsafe, but it can also come from your second chakra, which reflects your emotional state, and from your third chakra, when you take on too much and suddenly feel overwhelmed, like you just don't have the inner resources or personal power to deal with everything.

In other words, anxiety is a chakra one-two-three problem. Even if you aren't sure why you are feeling anxious or can't calm down, try this exercise, for a security/emotional/power boost that will help you let go of the anxiety and relax.

Don't panic! Try this exercise whenever you feel super stressed, overwhelmed, anxious, or panicky. Be sure to do this exercise in a quiet place where you won't be disturbed for at least five minutes by family members, friends, pets, the telephone, or the sound of your computer telling you that you have a new message.

1. Sit on the floor, on the edge of a folded blanket. Sit straight, as if you were rising up from the crown of your head. Pull your entire torso up, as if making space between each vertebra in your spine. Feel a lift in your chest and at the crown of your head, but keep your tailbone tucked in and down.

2. Visualize your first three chakras: the red chakra at the base of your spine, the orange chakra at your navel, and the yellow chakra just below your breastbone. Imagine each of them, glowing in their separate bright, clear colors.

3. Now, imagine each chakra getting bigger and radiating so that its circle merges with the others. Red becomes orange, orange becomes yellow, yellow becomes orange, orange becomes red, until each individual chakra dissolves into one bright glowing super chakra that encompasses your entire lower body.

4. Visualize this super chakra turning faster, until it begins to generate suction, like a funnel. See each individual worry, anxious thought, and panicky feeling getting sucked into this funnel and funneled out beyond the perimeter of your physical body. As it continues to spin and suck out anxious feelings like a vacuum, imagine this super chakra getting larger and stronger, radiating and forming a secure shield around your body that keeps those extracted feelings out.

5. Now, imagine this super chakra expanding, encompassing all your other chakras and reaching beyond the boundaries of your physical body until it encloses you in a safe, secure, warm, private space. The super chakra expands by pushing individual thoughts even farther back so you can still see them but they do not activate your mind into a worried state. You stand in the middle of this super chakra, calm, clear, and quiet, with an objective view of your external situation. Let ideas come to you, but not worries or scenarios about the future, which aren't allowed into this sacred space.

6. Continue to exist in this expanded space created by your first three chakras until you feel calm. During this time, you may suddenly know what to do to improve your situation. Or you will feel calm enough to move ahead without worry because your first three chakras have helped you put things into perspective.

7. Repeat whenever anxiety builds up again.

Courage comes from your first and third chakras, where you project your feelings of security and personal power. Your chakra power can ground you and light the way, so you can accomplish almost anything without fear stopping you.

Whenever you feel fearful or nervous or are trying to get yourself to do something brave (whether getting up in front of an audience to speak, playing your guitar at a party, or confronting someone with a difficult truth), try this easy exercise. You can do this wherever you are and whatever you are doing.

Visualize your deep red strong Root chakra anchoring you to the earth like a massive network of thick heavy unassailable tree roots reaching straight down into the earth.

At the same time, picture your third chakra radiating like a brilliant sun from just below your breastbone, blinding everyone with power, strength, and the light of truth.

Master of Concentration

Everybody has trouble concentrating once in a while, but sometimes concentration is crucial. When that happens, tap into the energy in your Throat and Third Eye chakras, the centers for communication, creativity, thought, and understanding.

The combined power of the fifth and sixth chakras can bring clarity and focus to anything you do, not to mention a creative spark that can carry your work, play, or interaction with others to new levels of brilliance.

To amp up your focus, you just need a warm-up, like stretching before a workout at the gym. *Dharana* is one of the Eight Limbs of Yoga, and it means concentration. Try this mini *dharana* exercise, and then turn your newfound focus to the task at hand. You'll be amazed at how well this works.

1. Sit quietly anywhere. A seat at your desk is just as good as a seat on a yoga mat. Sit up straight so you are not leaning back against anything. Relax.

2. Look around and find some small thing to look at. This can be anything small, like the eraser on a pencil, a flower petal, a letter on a piece of paper, or the power button on your computer. Center your attention on this visual point of focus.

3. Imagine a deep indigo beam radiating from your Third Eye chakra and hitting this object. At the same time, imagine a bright blue beam radiating from your Throat chakra and hitting this object. Let indigo-blue light surround the object and imagine sending energy through these beams to the object. Imagine the energy circulating back, as if the object is beaming it or reflecting it back to you.

4. Stay focused on this object for just one or two minutes. Now, get to work!

Weight Loss Made Easy

Okay, disclaimer: weight loss isn't easy. However, chakra power can make it easier than it would be without. That's because *agni*, the digestive fire, resides inside your third chakra. This is the seat of digestion and metabolism. When *agni* is stoked, you burn your food and fuel rather than storing it as fat.

However, becoming overweight also tends to be a function of the second chakra—many people overeat because of emotional reasons rather than pure physical hunger. Using food to pacify or smother strong feelings is pretty common, especially among people who are overweight. Process emotions in a healthy way by opening the second chakra, and you won't need to try to smother them.

If you need to lose weight, spend time reading the chapters on the second and third chakra, and do all the exercises for activating, aligning, and balancing these chakras. Losing weight takes a while and works only if you change the habits that caused you to gain weight in the first place. Temporary diets usually result in weight gain after the diet ends.

We could write a whole book on using the chakras for weight loss (and maybe we will someday), but for now, we will tell you that if you make it a habit to do a once-daily

Passion-Power chakra balance, you will stoke your digestive fire, feel more personally empowered, and find yourself better able to manage strong feelings so you don't keep turning to food when you aren't really hungry. When you do eat, this exercise will also help you burn that fuel faster. You might feel warmer after doing this exercise, but that's a good thing. Your metabolism and your motivation are stoked.

Practice this exercise once a day, before your first meal or before your largest meal. This exercise is based on a yoga *pranayama* exercise called *bhastrika*, often called Bellows Breath. Don't go too fast before you get used to this exercise, or you could hyperventilate. Don't do this exercise before bed, or you might have trouble sleeping. With regular practice, you will increase your metabolism and also build your abdominal strength.

def•i•ni•tion

Bhastrika is a yoga *pranayama* exercise involving quick exhalations to stoke the body's inner fire. Doing too much *bhasktrika* before the body is used to it could cause hyperventilation, so start slowly.

Energy Unplugged

Increase your inner fire even more effectively by spicing your foods with warming spices like ginger, cinnamon, cumin, turmeric, red pepper, and black pepper. Before bed, relax with a cup of warm milk (soy milk works, too) with a dash each of ginger, cinnamon, and turmeric, or enjoy ginger or cinnamon tea.

1. Sit comfortably on the floor, on the edge of a folded blanket. Cross your legs. Rest your hands on your knees.

2. Envision your second chakra as a bright clear orange light behind your navel, and your third chakra as a bright clear yellow light just under your rib cage. Imagine both lights growing brighter.

3. Now, imagine a tiny flame right between your second and third chakras. This flame is small but bright and active, with tongues of orange and yellow.

4. Pretend you are going to blow on this flame to make it brighter and stronger. At the count of one second per inhalation and one second per exhalation, begin breathing in rhythm through your nose, in and out, in and out.

5. Slowly increase the force and sound of your exhalation, so that you inhale silently but exhale sharply with a *HHM* or *HA* sound while tightening your abdominal muscles to help force out the air. (You might need a tissue!)

Exhale sharply when practicing Bellows Breath.

6. Repeat this inhale-exhale 10 to 20 times. Every time you exhale, imagine the inner flame getting brighter, larger, and hotter.

7. Repeat once each day, adding a few more breaths each day until you work up to 100. Don't go too quickly, though. It should take you at least one month to reach 100 of these breaths.

8. Enjoy increased metabolism, more inner fire, more confidence and strength, and slow, gradual, healthy weight loss.

The Least You Need to Know

♦ You can use the different kinds of energy within each chakra to address different kinds of issues in your life.

♦ Chakra work feels good not only because it balances the energy in your body but because it turns your focus inward, forcing you to pay attention to your own needs, and can actually help heal physical and emotional problems.

♦ Combining the energies within multiple chakras can effectively address specific problems, such as insomnia, pain, anxiety, fearfulness, and concentration problems.

♦ Working with your chakras can help you lose excess weight more easily.

Toning: Singing the Body Chakra

In This Chapter

- Toning your chakras with your own voice
- Finding your own vibration
- Sacred syllables
- Vowel power
- Toning improvisation
- Chanting and mantra meditation

You are energy. You vibrate with it, and it flows through you. Without it, you would not be alive. Energy is the spark that illuminates and animates you, and one of the main ways we feel that energy is by feeling its vibration.

Our chakras spin as energy moves through them and around them, transforming energy in different ways according to which chakra pulls in that energy and then moves it back out through the body. Chakras change with each passing moment and each new experience, but sometimes they get stuck. They close down to protect themselves, or get so flooded with energy that they suck all the energy from the chakras above and below, throwing the body's functioning out of whack. When this happens, the body's vibrations get out of tune, but you can use your chakras to correct that imbalance. That's what this chapter is all about.

Good Vibrations

Sound is an incredibly powerful tool for tuning up the chakras. This is called *toning* (rather than tuning). This sound can come from a tuning fork or instrument, but it can also come from your own voice.

If you've ever sung in a choir or even with just one other person, you may know what it is like to be unsure of a note until you hear it. Then, when someone else sings it, your voice slides right into tune alongside the other voice. The vibration of that other voice has coaxed your vibration along with it until the two voices merge.

In much the same way, creating the vibration of a chakra with your voice can nudge an out-of-tune chakra back into its natural vibration. This sympathetic vibration is an excellent way to bring the chakras back into tune and help energy to flow more freely through them. This, in turn, leads to healing, as each chakra vibrates according to its own nature.

def•i•ni•tion

Toning is a technique for balancing, energizing, and strengthening the chakras using sound, particularly the sound of your own voice. Toning techniques may employ vowel sounds, sacred syllables associated with each chakra, or improvisational vocalizations.

You can start singing right now if you want to, but first, let's talk about making sound, and what that means to you. We've read a lot of things about toning and chanting, and we've tried a lot of those things for ourselves, to see what works and what doesn't. Each chakra has a sacred syllable, a vowel sound that activates it, and certain sounds that resonate within it. However, what those syllables, vowels, and sounds are varies depending on who you ask.

As far as *you* are concerned, we strongly suggest that you find the sounds that resonate with you. When you make any sound with your voice, you can direct that sound to any part of your body and it can resonate, so choose the sounds that feel most natural and right.

For example, is the vowel associated with the Root chakra the sound of *uh*, as in cup, or *oh*, as in soap? Different sources tell you different things, so try them both and see which one resonates most within your first chakra. If you can't tell, then choose the one you like best. It doesn't matter why you like it, just pick the sound that makes you feel good. Your intention and how you decide to use the sounds are arguably more important than what sounds you use.

Much of this chapter involves making sounds that are intuitive. What if you just started making sounds? Would you be wrong? No. What comes out of your body is what your body produces, and that is what is right for your body.

However, you can learn to tone in a way that increases vibration more efficiently, so before we get into the different sounds associated with each chakra, let's practice a little.

You remember learning the vowels in school, right? A, E, I, O, U, and sometimes Y? Let's start there. Don't worry about what these sounds do right now. Just practice making sounds.

> **!!! Wake-Up Call** _____
>
> Some people vocalize with ease, while for others, vocalizing doesn't come easily at all. In the latter case, the problem is likely in the fifth chakra. This chakra is the center of communication, speaking, listening, music, and sound. This is where you make noise. You groan, giggle, sigh, and sing from your fifth chakra. If this chakra is blocked, you may feel very uncomfortable vocalizing, especially randomly without specific directions. If this sounds like you, skip back to Chapter 11 on the fifth chakra and try the exercises for energizing, aligning, and balancing this important source of sound in your body. Then come back to this chapter and try again. You may need to spend some time finding your own voice, but almost everybody can learn to vocalize, so give yourself a chance to develop your innate vocal talents.

Make Noise

Are you ready to make some noise?

If you feel self-conscious, you might want to try this when you are home alone or in a room where nobody can hear you. Don't feel silly. Making sound is one of your own body's most joyful acts and powerful healing tools.

First, sit on the floor or on a chair with your spine straight. You need plenty of space inside your torso for the sound to resonate, so don't slump against a backrest. If it's more comfortable, you can also stand.

Now, say the letter A, as in "say." Just say it once. Hear your voice. Notice the pitch. Say it again and hold it longer. Try to feel it vibrating inside your body. You will feel it in your throat, but where else do you feel it? Does the vibration want to settle somewhere?

Try saying it at a lower pitch, or a higher pitch. Move it around. Don't worry if it doesn't sound "good." You aren't trying out for *American Idol*. Just make the sound. Get used to the feel of your own voice making that sound: *AAAAAAAYYYYYY*. Notice what the vibration of that sound does inside your body.

As you practice, notice how you can make the sound in a pinched, tight way that doesn't vibrate very much, or in a deep, resonant way that vibrates more. The more resonant the sound is, the better. The more you practice, the more you will get the hang of making a deep, vibrating sound. Don't be intimidated or shy. Try to just let it loose. Open up and relax your throat. Put more breath behind the sound. Try it louder, or softer. You can even be silly. Make wavy sounds or zig-zag sounds. Just make sounds.

Most importantly, feel which sounds seem most right, true, and resonant within *you*.

Fun with Vowels

After you've moved your AY sound around and tried it in lots of different ways, go to the next vowel: E. Try that sound: *EEEEEE*. Experiment with different pitches, volume, and vibrations. Notice where you feel this sound in your body. Is it different than when you said *AAAYYY*?

After you've played around with EE for a while, move on to the rest of the vowels: I (*AYE*), O (*OH*), and U (*YOU*).

Keep practicing, and if you feel compelled to make other noises, whether vowels or consonants or suddenly breaking into that song you always hear on the radio, go ahead! The point is to set your voice free.

The other point is to determine what sounds make sense to your body and your chakras. Because your chakras are unique to you and your voice and vibrations are unique to you, too, different sounds will work better for you than others.

You have to tune in to your voice and the way your body feels to determine this, however, so if you still feel unsure about the sounds that resonate with you, don't let it hold you back. Keep practicing, keep using your intuition and your feelings, and your toning skills will quickly improve.

Spinning Your Wheels

Our favorite sound specialist, Joseph Mizelle, is a licensed massage therapist, certified yoga teacher, and sound energy healer who works at the Eastwind Healing Center in Iowa City, Iowa, where Betsy has her practice. One of the techniques Joseph uses is to actually vocalize into the chakras of his clients. This incredibly powerful technique shows that someone else's vibrations can influence yours. For example, if Joseph is giving someone a massage and recognizes tightness or a block in a certain area, he will vocalize using his deep, incredibly (almost unbelievably) resonant voice, right above the chakra. This could be in the lower back or neck or wherever the problem is. The person receiving the vibration can actually feel it pretty intensely, like a buzzing, inside that chakra. Joseph says that some people experience incredible emotional release during a sound healing session, and many of his clients say that the session takes them to some pretty amazing places. If you have a sound healer near you, you might want to try a session.

Speaking Chakra

Traditionally, each of the seven primary chakras has a seed sound associated with it. Sometimes you will see this sound written as (to use the first chakra as an example) *LAM*. In other places, you will see it written as *LANG*, which is the Tibetan version. Because your chakras are unique to you and your voice and vibrations are unique to you, too, you may prefer one or the other. It's up to you.

Now that you have warmed up, you can start experimenting with these seed sounds for each chakra. We've listed all the seed sounds in the following chart, for easy reference. All sounds rhyme with *mom* or *song*, except *OM*, which rhymes more closely with *home*, and the seventh chakra, which has no rhyme.

Chakra	Seed Sound	Rhymes with
First/Root chakra	*LANG*	Mom or Song
Second/Passion chakra	*VANG*	Mom or Song
Third/Solar Plexus chakra	*RANG*	Mom or Song
Fourth/Heart chakra	*YANG*	Mom or Song
Fifth/Throat chakra	*HANG*	Mom or Song
Sixth/Third Eye chakra	*OM (AUM)* or *ANG*	Home or Song
Seventh/Crown chakra	*NNG* or no sound (listen)	Home or Song

To practice using these sounds, try this exercise. We use the first seed sound listed in the previous chart (such as *LAM* or VAM) instead of the second (such as *LANG* or *VANG*), but you can use either one:

1. Sit on the floor on the edge of a folded blanket. Sit up straight to make room inside your chest.

2. Bring your attention to your first chakra. Visualize a red wheel turning slowly at the base of your spine. Take a deep breath, then say *LAM*, holding the vowel for as long as you can, but leaving enough breath to let the final consonant vibrate.

3. Inhale as you bring your attention to your second chakra. Visualize an orange wheel turning slowly in your abdomen just behind your navel. Say *VAM*, holding the vowel for as long as you can, but leaving enough breath to let the final consonant vibrate.

4. Inhale as you bring your attention to your third chakra. Visualize a yellow wheel turning slowly just beneath your rib cage at your solar plexus. Say *RAM*, holding the vowel for as long as you can, but leaving enough breath to let the final consonant vibrate.

5. Inhale as you bring your attention to your fourth chakra. Visualize a green wheel turning slowly around your heart. Say *YAM*, holding the vowel for as long as you can, but leaving enough breath to let the final consonant vibrate.

6. Inhale as you bring your attention to your fifth chakra. Visualize a blue wheel turning slowly just above your collarbone in your throat. Say *HAM*, holding the vowel for as long as you can, but leaving enough breath to let the final consonant vibrate.

7. Inhale as you bring your attention to your sixth chakra. Visualize an indigo or purple wheel turning slowly in the middle of your forehead. Say *OM*, holding the vowel for as long as you can, but leaving enough breath to let the final consonant vibrate.

8. Inhale as you bring your attention to your seventh chakra. Visualize a purple or white wheel turning slowly just above the crown of your head. Say *NNG* (like the final two consonants in the word *sing*), holding the sound for as long as you can, but leaving enough breath to let the final consonant vibrate. Or just listen during this breath. The seed sound of this chakra is traditionally the universe vibrating with the sound of *OM*, with no sound from you at all.

The Sanskrit symbol for OM.

![Energy Unplugged]

Energy Unplugged

When vocalizing sounds or vowels for each chakra, the usual technique is to start with a low voice when focusing on the first chakra, and gradually raise the pitch so that the vocalization for the seventh chakra is the highest pitch of all. This might not work well for you, but try it to see if it makes sense and resonates with your chakras.

The Power of the Vowel

Although any sound can resonate inside the body, vowels seem to have a particular vibration that easily energizes the chakras. In his book *Healing Sounds*, author Jonathan Goldman says one of the reasons he likes to use vowels for chakra healing is that they are not words in other languages that people may find unfamiliar, or that may make people uncomfortable, especially if they practice a particular religion and don't want to chant words that they feel are associated with a different religion. Motivation aside, vowels do resonate particularly well within the body and are an excellent way to tone the chakras.

As we mentioned in the beginning of this chapter, however, there are different systems that apply different vowel sounds to each chakra. In this book, we show you one of the more common systems, but if other vowels work better for activating your own chakras, you can certainly use those.

To tone your chakras with vowel sounds, practice the same way you practiced speaking the seed sounds in the previous section, but use these vowels as you focus on each chakra, one at a time.

Start by doing one vowel sound per breath for each chakra, as in the previous exercise. Or concentrate on a single chakra that you think needs some work, and repeat that vowel sound over and over as you keep your attention focused on the appropriate chakra. When you do this, your vowel sound becomes a sort of *mantra*.

def•i•ni•tion

Mantra is the Sanskrit word for a sacred syllable or phrase that is spoken repeatedly during meditation, to aid in concentration and focus.

The following chart contains some of the sounds you can use. These are common vowel sounds associated with each chakra, and also the ones that resonate best with us.

Chakra	Vowel Sound	The Same Vowel Sound As
First/Root chakra	UH	Sun
Second/Passion chakra	OO	Shoe
Third/Solar Plexus chakra	OH	Slow
Fourth/Heart chakra	AH	Saw
Fifth/Throat chakra	EYE	Sigh
Sixth/Third Eye chakra	AY	Say
Seventh/Crown chakra	EE	See

Chakra Scat Singing

With regular practice, you will soon become familiar with speaking seed sounds and toning vowels to tone your chakras and get your energy flowing, but you can go even further. Try vocalizing according to your intuition. Make sounds—any sounds—that don't necessarily involve the formation of words.

Let your feelings flow from your voice and communicate themselves through vibration rather than logical language sense. Having a strong, balanced, open fifth chakra helps, but even if you are having problems with your own personal communication skills, you can still try this. In fact, it might be enough to open that fifth chakra right up. Have fun with this. It doesn't have to be serious. Make sounds that fill you with joy.

Spinning Your Wheels

Eve loves to vocalize, and when she isn't writing books, she is sometimes singing with her father's jazz band. Occasionally, they play at a nearby casino, and Eve's dad likes to joke that all the slot machines are ringing in the key of C. Actually, musical notes are associated with each chakra, and it's ironic that the slot machines would play C because C is associated with the first chakra, which is the chakra associated with financial security. Maybe that constant C sound influences people to believe that playing those slots will ensure wealth. If only it were so! The second/Passion chakra's note is D, the third/Power chakra's note is E, the fourth/Heart chakra's note is F, the fifth/Throat chakra's note is G, the sixth/Third Eye chakra's note is A, and the seventh/Crown chakra's note is B.

Random vocalization can be difficult. You might be wondering what the heck you are supposed to be saying. Don't worry about that. We've heard beautiful solos by vocalists who just made sounds according to their intuition at the moment. In fact, that's what jazz scat singing is. But you don't have to sound like Ella Fitzgerald. Just make sound. Start with an AHH or an OHH or an OOH or an EEE. See where it goes.

Vocalizing according to your intuition can free up your inner voice. Pay attention to what noise you want to make, and honor it. Let yourself sing, and your chakras will respond. Nobody has to hear it but you.

Chanting and Mantra Meditation

One of the most common ways to use sound and vocalization as it relates to the chakras is through chanting and *mantra meditation*. We left this section for the end because we wanted to focus on more basic techniques first, but even if you don't like toning, you might enjoy meditating using mantras.

Mantra meditation is a form of meditation that involves chanting a mantra repeatedly, as an anchor or focus for meditation. This keeps the mind centered on one point and the vibration from the chanting can also alter the course of the meditation in interesting ways. To practice mantra meditation, you can use any of the seed sounds or vowel sounds in this chapter. Sit quietly and repeat the sounds, either outloud for maximum vibration power or just in your mind, and let these sounds anchor your awareness.

You can also chant when you aren't meditating. Many yoga classes begin with particular chants, like prayers, to set the right intention and mood. When people get together to chant, it is called *kirtan* in India. Musicians typically play and sing chants and the people participating in the *kirtan* repeat the chants in a call-and-response format. Some people chant at home as part of a daily ritual.

So make some sound, whether you are meditating or chanting or working with a particular chakra or just celebrating a beautiful day. Let your body vibrate with sound. You have a sacred instrument within you that has the power to tune up your chakras and get your energy flowing again. We hope this chapter has helped you discover how to begin using that instrument, for healthier chakras and a more joyful life.

The Least You Need to Know

- ◆ Toning is a way to balance and heal chakras using sound. By singing or playing the correct vibration, the chakra returns to its natural state.

- ◆ Each chakra has a traditional seed sound and vowel sound that energizes and tunes it, but the particular sounds and vowels you might use to tone your chakras can vary, depending on what sounds resonate best with your own body and your chakras.

- ◆ Freestyle vocalization is good therapy for your fifth chakra and all your chakras. Let your voice ring out and let the good vibrations flow through your body, healing your chakras and bringing you joy.

Chapter 16

Tantra: Chakras and Love

In This Chapter

- ◆ Tantra truths and myths
- ◆ Sex and the Heart chakra
- ◆ Sex and the Passion chakra
- ◆ Initiating your own divine union

Now for the fun part. Not that the rest of it hasn't been fun, but now we're talking *fun*. In other words, we're talking sex.

Sex is about pleasure, fulfillment, and most importantly, about connection, and because these are all aspects directly reflected in the chakras, working with the chakras can enhance and intensify your sexual experience. Chakras: the ultimate relationship aid!

When you look to the chakras to improve your sexual experience, you will quickly understand that this approach takes sex beyond the physical. The idea that sex is a spiritual act is nothing new. Sex as a metaphor for union with the divine universal spirit is ancient and a part of many different traditions. Hinduism explores this metaphor. So does Taoism in China, many of the ancient pagan religions from Europe, and even Christianity, where nuns marry God. In all these traditions, however, sexual energy is transformed into spiritual energy, rather than being "wasted" on plain old physical kicks.

But maybe you didn't sign up for some esoteric spiritual experience. You just want to get healthy, feel good, and have better sex. No problem. We can help you with that. However, to do so, we need a brief lesson in Tantra.

The Truth About Tantra

The tradition that is relevant for this chapter is *Tantra*. Talking about sex in a book about chakras pretty much demands discussing Tantra, even though understanding Tantric philosophy can be the work of an entire lifetime. But we promise to keep things simple.

def•i•ni•tion

Tantra is a branch of the yoga tradition often associated with sexual practices, but this is a misunderstanding of this esoteric form of yoga. According to Tantra, our sensory experience and the physical universe itself is a manifestation of divine energy, and so should be celebrated, rather than transcended.

Tantra is a school of yogic thought that arose as a backlash against the traditional philosophy that the material world, including the body, is illusory and distracting, a source of suffering, and that it must be transcended in order to experience enlightenment. Tantra says no! According to Tantric thought, the world is beautiful, the body is beautiful, and physical pleasure is beautiful, too. In fact, the physical universe, including the body, is a manifestation of divine perfection, so enjoying and celebrating these things is just like worship. Isn't that nice?

Tantra is nice, but it also has a naughty reputation. People automatically associate Tantra with sex and esoteric sexual rituals. Sexual rituals are a part of Tantra, it's true. However, they are just one part, a very advanced part, and definitely not the *point* of Tantra.

Spinning Your Wheels

Despite what you may have heard, the *Kama Sutra* has nothing to do with Tantra and never mentions the chakras. The *Kama Sutra* is a practical treatise on sexual techniques and the art of love, penned by a Hindu scholar named Vatsyayana in about the fourth century and translated for English audiences in the 1800s by an Englishman named Sir Richard Burton. It is meant to guide, instruct, and counsel a sexual society on everything from handling multiple wives to kissing to the best ways to stimulate the clitoris. You can certainly use some of the techniques in the *Kama Sutra* as you seek to have a deeper sexual relationship, but don't mistake the *Kama Sutra* for a Tantric text.

Tantra means "weaving together," and the Tantric philosophy says fulfillment comes through the weaving together of opposites: heaven and Earth, day and night, sun and moon, and of course, male and female.

The Tantric philosophy of the universe is that (to simplify) there are two divine parents, not just one male god or female goddess. There is the divine feminine and the divine masculine. The divine feminine is earthy, unruly, dark, wild, full of movement, even a little dangerous. The divine masculine is steady, bright, serene, and infused with spirit. Each is amazing and fantastic and fascinating, but neither is whole without the other. Wild earthy movement is steadied by bright serene spirit, and bright serene spirit is enlivened and animated by wild earthy movement. Doesn't that sound sexy?

Tantric philosophy also involves *Kundalini*. We go into more detail about *Kundalini* in Chapter 5, and if you read that chapter already, you probably remember that *Kundalini* is latent, powerful, wild, unruly, feminine energy that waits inside the first chakra to be awakened. When *Kundalini* awakens, she seeks her mate, the serene spiritual male energy. She moves up through the seven chakras, as each is ready to receive her, piercing them as she rises to the Crown chakra where she can finally unite in divine union with her male counterpart, who is frequently represented, in Hindu literature, as the god Shiva.

We think that's pretty sexy, too, and in Tantra, that's just what sex is—a sort of acting out of this divine partnership, where male and female join together in ecstatic union that is both intensely pleasurable and significantly spiritual—the best of both worlds.

What Tantra Isn't

Knowing what you now know about Tantra, it is probably pretty clear that some of the ideas people have about Tantra aren't true. Tantra is not about new complicated sexual positions or role playing or having multiple sex partners.

Tantra is not just sex, sex, sex, either. In fact, most Tantric rituals don't even involve sex. They are about connection, about weaving together opposites, and about union in all its many forms. Yes, Tantra can increase your physical and sexual energy, but also channels that energy in a way that increases pleasure, joy, and bonding.

Tantra isn't actually a religion, either. It is a philosophy. If you sign up for a Tantra yoga class, we can guarantee you that you won't be rolling around having sex with the person on the mat next to yours. Tantra is about opening up your mind and body to experience divine or universal energy in order to comprehend the truth that we are all part of one great energetic body. There are many ways to do that. Sex is just one of them.

> ## (!!!) Wake-Up Call
>
> If you have a same-sex partner, never fear. You can still experience sacred sex. Each human being has a mixture of feminine and masculine qualities that seek each other. When you and your partner become immersed in the passionate energy of sexual union, all those energies will find each other, and the merging will be just as explosive. Your technical physical parts don't matter one bit.

The Heart Chakra: Your Sexual Command Center

You may recall from Chapter 8 that the second chakra, sometimes called the Passion chakra or Sexual chakra, is the chakra that reflects our sexual desires, pleasures, and longings. That's true, and we'll get to the second chakra in the next section. However, when it comes to sex and the chakras (doesn't that sound like some new HBO series?), the fourth chakra, or Heart chakra, really is your sexual command center.

Remember how *Kundalini* works? As wild, earthy, unruly *Kundalini* rises up toward the steady, bright, divine masculine, that steady bright divinity can't help being drawn downward toward earthy grounding pleasure, and guess where they meet? All that energy collides and explodes right in the middle chakra exactly between the three earthly chakras and the three heavenly chakras. Remember, Tantra means weaving and the union of opposites, and where else to merge those opposites than on neutral ground? The Heart chakra is that neutral ground.

When we talked about *Kundalini* before, you might remember that we talked about how it rises up through all seven chakras to find fulfillment at the Crown chakra. That's true, but it's also a bit of an oversimplification. *Kundalini* does seek to rise all the way up through each chakra, but divine energy is always seeking the earth, too, so the person with seven open, balanced chakras experiences all kinds of back and forth, up and down energy.

Although not all sources agree on this, we subscribe to the notion that *Kundalini* can rise up, then fall down, then rise up again, just as divine energy can radiate all the way down from the Crown to the Root chakra, then flow back up. Our bodies and indeed our chakras are vessels for our own constantly fluctuating and circulating energies, both masculine and feminine, earthy and spiritual. Where the real combustion happens during sexual union, however, is in the Heart chakra.

That means if you have a blocked Heart chakra, you might experience isolation during sexual intercourse, rather than union. You might also experience personal pleasure, but feel nothing for the person helping to provide this pleasure.

During sex, your body does everything it can to orgasm so that chemicals can be released that promote bonding. However, a blocked Heart chakra can reroute those pleasurable feelings so you begin to associate them not with the other person but only with yourself. When sexual pleasure becomes purely self-centered, sexual addiction can be the result—a constant search for the pleasure, rush, and "high" of sex without any feelings linked to the sexual partner.

Spinning Your Wheels

One of Tantra's more talked-about techniques involves the notion that if orgasm can be suppressed, sexual energy will move back up toward the Crown chakra, rather than out of the body. The theory goes that sexual energy is so potent and powerful that releasing it through orgasm wastes it on mere physical pleasure. Instead, by becoming aroused and then directing the energy up through the *sushumna nadi* towards the Crown chakra, all that potent energy stays within the body and moves the consciousness closer to enlightenment, which is the ultimate ecstasy.

Seeking sex for pure personal pleasure is a hard problem to address because there is typically little motivation to change this behavior when the sex seeker sees few negative consequences. However, that is only because the person with the blocked Heart chakra has not experienced the much more intense, much more pleasurable and complete experience of sexual pleasure that is based in total spiritual union rather than shallow physical pleasure.

Sex and the Passion Chakra

But let's not forget the second chakra, where all that pleasure begins. Masculine and feminine energy may meet at the Heart chakra, but the physical, earthy, sensual-pleasure part of sex comes from the second chakra.

If the second chakra is blocked, it becomes difficult to experience physical pleasure during sex, and this physical pleasure—and all its associated chemical signals in the body—is an intrinsic part of the sexual experience. The second chakra also reflects the body's fertility and creativity, which sexual energy can illuminate. A closed second chakra blocks off all those other wonderful, rich aspects of sexual union.

Remember that in Tantra, physical pleasure is a manifestation of divine ecstasy. It is not something to feel guilty about. It is something to celebrate, honor, and revel in, as you join totally with another human being. Without it, sex is just an exercise, like doing sit-ups.

An overloaded second chakra can get in the way of sexual pleasure, too. The second chakra is the source of feelings, emotions, and passions. Get too needy, too clingy, or too desperate because of an overloaded second chakra, and the whole experience goes out of balance. This overload may also lead to engaging in sex purely out of self-ish reasons. If you feel empty inside, you may believe merging sexually with another will fill your cup. It may, in the moment, but when the event is over, the emptiness returns. Ideally, sexual union is about the merging of equally potent energies, and if you can fill yourself up without needing someone else to do this task, sex can reach the next level of true connection and ecstasy.

Ideally, when the Passion chakra is open, balanced, and strong, the physical arousal and pleasure you will get from sexual union will be enough to make you weak in the knees. When your Heart chakra is open, balanced, and strong as well, you'll have plenty of inner space for masculine and feminine energies to merge into one complete and realized whole as your body merges with another body that is experiencing the same thing. Two become one, and that is sacred.

Energy Unplugged

The second chakra is located just above the genitals. An exercise to help open and energize the second chakra is to get very close to your partner and press your second chakras together—abdomen to abdomen. (You can be clothed, or not.) Stay in this position for a full five minutes, looking at each other directly in the eyes (which also opens the Heart chakra). Don't speak or move. (Giggling may be unavoidable.) This is an intense exercise and more difficult than it sounds, but can really get that Passion chakra energy flowing.

Can't All the Chakras Have Some Fun?

Kundalini energy can't move up the spine seeking her masculine counterpart if any of the chakra doors are slammed shut, and each and every chakra does play its own role in the sexual experience. The more open and balanced all your chakras, the more complete your union will be.

Regular chakra work, regular yoga, regular massage, and yes, regular sex with a loving partner will all contribute to healthy, open chakras, but as further motivation, here are each chakra's contributions to your great sex experience:

◆ The healthy first chakra makes you feel secure enough that you can reach out to another human being without feeling like your own identity is at risk. The first chakra also takes care of your basic needs so you don't have to worry about the unpaid electric bill or getting enough to eat when you are trying to focus on more elevated pleasures.

◆ The healthy second chakra provides actual pleasurable sensations within the body, the ability to feel your own body and the body of someone else, and a steady emotional connection with your partner. Swellings of passionate feeling and the desire to reach out and merge with another body also come from here.

◆ The healthy third chakra gives sexual union power and volatility. It is the part of you that recognizes yourself as an individual, and the other person as a different individual. It is also the part that gives you the courage and fortitude to step forward and extend a metaphorical hand to another human being, which isn't always easy to do.

◆ The healthy fourth chakra serves as the energetic "bed" on which feminine and masculine energies consummate their union. This exact center of the chakras is the meeting ground for Earth and heaven, and it also enhances sexual union with sensitivity, compassion, sacrifice, the desire to please someone other than yourself, and ultimately, love that far exceeds pure physical sensation.

◆ The healthy fifth chakra provides a mental context for physical union. This is where we understand what sex is, as well as what it means. We speak to our partners from here, but we also listen, not just to the other's words but to actions, movements, and expressions. Without this capacity, sex withdraws into the purely physical without understanding of its implications, without a true understanding of the other person, and without any heightened sense of the meaning of union.

◆ The healthy sixth chakra adds subtlety and nuance to the sexual experience. Without intuition, sex can become basic and desensitized, but with the health of the sixth chakra, each partner becomes keenly aware of what the other needs. This kind of mutual awareness catapults sex out of the realm of the ordinary or of duty to make it an art form. The sixth chakra adds the embroidered details to the Tantric weaving.

◆ The healthy seventh chakra brings sex out of the physical world and adds the final universal dimension that makes sex not just pleasurable but divine. With seventh chakra involvement, sex is still a union of two bodies, but it also represents the union of body and spirit, of heaven and Earth, and of the human with the divine.

Chakra Bonding for Better Sex

So how can *you* have yourself some sacred sex? Try these Tantric-inspired techniques, some to try with your partner and some just for you, and remember, practice makes perfect!

Down-Under Workouts for Greater Orgasmic Control

You can't run a marathon without getting in shape and you can't expect to have an intense prolonged sexual experience without getting in shape, either. Yet, to build up sexual energy for a more complete and total merging experience, you can't just rush through sex and fall asleep. You need to take some time.

But that takes stamina and the ability to control the rush to pleasure. Regular cardio-vascular exercise actually goes a long way toward improving sexual endurance. It also improves body image so you will be less inhibited, have more fun, and maybe even experience more intense pleasure from sex.

However, you can also spot-train for better sex and better orgasmic control. Both men and women have muscles around their sexual organs and pelvic floor that help to control and sustain orgasms. If you tend to be highly orgasmic and reach orgasm too quickly, toning these muscles can help you control that rush to pleasure. If you have trouble having an orgasm at all, toning these muscles can finally make the Big O a reality in your life.

To begin conditioning this area, squeeze the pelvic floor muscles and release them in a pulsing movement. This is the same muscular contraction you would use to stop the flow of urine. (This applies to both men and women.) These are sometimes called Kegel exercises.

Once you get the feel of it, do 10 repetitions. A few hours later, do it again. If you can do this a few times a day and gradually work up to about 50 reps, your muscles will be in great shape for whatever challenges they might encounter.

Shakti and Shiva

Sometimes husbands, wives, boyfriends, girlfriends, can be so ... *annoying*. They don't load the dishwasher the right way or they forget to put gas in the car. They have that little habit that just drives you *crazy*. But guess what? As much as your partner is a faulty and sometimes irritating human, he or she is also a God or Goddess.

We're not talking about idol worship here. We're not even talking about religion. We are talking about union because you are also a God or Goddess, the embodiment of divine energy. When it comes to sex, you have to let all those annoying things go. What's more, you have to ... or shall we say you *get to* ... worship your partner for the divine embodiment he or she truly is.

This brings a whole new energy to sexual union, one that can completely transform your relationship. If your first reaction is something to the effect of, "You want me to worship him? I don't think so!" or "Worship her? Don't I do enough for her already?" then we have news for you. You need to work on your Heart chakra.

Part of the potent power of sacred sexual union is in the merging of equal opposites, but the only way for that to happen is for both partners to open their hearts and fall down on their knees in worship of the other. It doesn't work if only one person does this, but if neither one will do it, if nobody wants to go first, then real union will never happen. One of the secrets of Shakti and Shiva is that mutual worship breaks down all barriers of separateness, ego, and the false idea that we are alone. If you worship your partner, your partner is likely to fall down in gratitude and worship you. This is human nature, and the beginning of an understanding of divine union. Although mutual worship probably won't be easy or fast-acting, when equal forces meet with open hearts and a sense of commitment, it can, and quite often will, turn into something beautiful.

Of Lingams and Yonis

Two of the sacred symbols of Tantra are the *lingam* and the *yoni*. The *lingam* is, essentially, a sacred phallic symbol that represents male energy. The *yoni* is the sacred symbol of the female sex organs, representing female energy. In ancient statues from India, these two symbols are often joined together and represent the energy that fuels the entire universe.

Another potent and energy-generating activity is to massage each other's *lingam* and *yoni* (take turns) without coming to orgasm. Focus on total relaxation. When excitement builds, stop. Wait. Then start again when the energy dies down. This gradual building up increases sexual energy to levels far beyond what can be achieved in regular sexual contact. Touch and worship your partner's *lingam* or *yoni*, but keep pulling back until the energy has built to a peak.

def•i•ni•tion

The *lingam* is an ancient symbol for male energy represented by a penis-like shape. The *yoni* is an ancient symbol for female energy represented by a vagina-like shape.

Ancient Hindu sculptures embrace the union of feminine (yoni) and masculine (lingam) energy.

We can't be responsible for what might happen next, but we hope you will keep exploring, keep coming together in union with your opposite, and keep worshipping the god and goddess in each other.

The Least You Need to Know

♦ Tantra is a yogic philosophy that embraces the physical world, the body, and physical pleasure as a manifestation of the divine rather than as something to be despised or transcended.

♦ Tantra means weaving together, and Tantric practices, although they include sexual rituals, are mostly not about sex. They are about unifying opposites, including the physical body's direct experience of divine energy.

♦ Although each chakra plays a part in sexual union of two people, the fourth or Heart chakra is where masculine and feminine energy meet, collide, and join, and the second or Passion chakra is where the body experiences physical pleasures and the emotional desire to merge with another. Keeping both these chakras open and healthy will enhance the sexual experience.

Chapter 17

Chakra Meditations

In This Chapter

- ◆ The power of chakra meditation
- ◆ Chakra meditation techniques explained
- ◆ Guided meditations for each of the seven chakras

As just about anybody who meditates regularly can tell you, meditation can be tough. It doesn't seem so hard, really. You just sit there, right? Counting your breaths and trying not to think, or something like that?

Actually, meditation means many different things, depending on which tradition you explore. Meditation can be sitting with an empty mind, or sitting with a completely mindful mind, or counting breaths, or chanting a mantra, or focusing on a visual point, or contemplating a question, or communing with God. It can happen while sitting or lying down or walking or dancing or laughing or spinning or making love.

It can also center around the chakras.

Chakra Meditation

Despite all the many techniques, meditation almost always has the same goal: to expand the boundaries of awareness until the mind moves beyond its individuality to experience unity with all things or with divine spirit. But most meditators can't just sit down and slip right into *samadhi*. They need some techniques to help get them there.

One of the most common and proven techniques is to focus the mind on one thing. This trains the mind to concentrate and helps combat scattered thinking and excessive mental chatter. In chakra meditation, the objects of contemplation, instead of a mantra to chant or an object to gaze upon, are the chakras.

Chakra meditation is incredibly relaxing, and also an excellent way for beginners to test the waters of meditation because it is a *guided meditation*. In a guided meditation, the meditation leader reads or speaks the meditation, leading the meditators through the steps. You don't have to try to clear your mind because you have someone else's voice and information on which to focus.

def•i•ni•tion

Samadhi is the last of the Eight Limbs of Yoga, as described by Patanjali in the *Yoga Sutras*. *Samadhi* is the direct experience of the unity of all things.

Guided meditation is a form of meditation in which someone reads or speaks the steps of a meditation, giving the people who are meditating a voice and a story or visualization to focus on. Guided meditation is an easy way to start learning how to meditate because it takes a little less discipline than just clearing the mind or focusing without anyone's help.

In particular, chakra meditation gives the mind something interesting, varied, beautiful, and self-involved to focus on—*way* more fun than just sitting there not thinking. As you get better at meditating on your own chakras, you can progress beyond hearing a guiding voice, meditating on your chakras without assistance.

Chakra Meditation How-To

Chakra meditation isn't difficult. However, it will be easier and more effective if you follow a few simple guidelines.

Who's Talking?

Obviously, you can't read these meditations out loud and also do the meditation at the same time. Instead, you could record your voice reading the meditations, then play them back (many cellular phones and mp3 players have voice recorders, or use an old-fashioned tape recorder).

Or ask someone to read or record the meditation for you. Once you are familiar with the meditation, you won't need to hear it anymore because you can just go through it in your head.

You can do the chakra meditations in this chapter separately, such as one per day, or you can do them all in one longer session. How long each will take depends on how fast you (or the person doing the reading) read the words and how much time you give to the pauses, but allow yourself about three to five minutes for each.

Set the Mood

Before you jump right in, set aside time during which you won't be disturbed by noise or interruptions, including the phone, children, or pets. Unplug or turn off your phone if necessary. Turn off the television and the computer. (It's only for 20 to 30 minutes if you do all the meditations.)

Find a place to meditate. Ideally, it should be a clean, uncluttered spot that relaxes you, but do the best you can. Choose the room that makes you feel the most relaxed. If it helps, drape sheets, scarves, or saris over clutter and turn down the lights. Many people find candlelight relaxing.

You can play relaxing mood music, too, but it should not contain any vocalizations. Turn the volume low enough that the music doesn't interfere with the sound of the voice guiding you through the meditation. Any music should enhance, not compete with, the meditation.

Energy Unplugged

We don't all have the luxury of a spare room or extra, unused space in our homes, but if you do, you might consider turning that spot into a meditation space. Keep your meditation space very clean and uncluttered with simple décor that makes you feel calm and peaceful. Many people with meditation areas set up an altar with items on it for meditative focus, such as candles, crystals, natural elements like shells or leaves, or pictures or statues of spiritual leaders or religious figures. Add a yoga mat and a folded blanket or meditation cushion. This room or space does *not* need a telephone or a television, but it can benefit from beautiful art, especially in the colors of the chakras that you most want to heal.

Getting Into Position

Sit or lie down in a position that keeps your spine straight and expanded. You don't want to be hunched over, twisted, or moving. The best positions are either:

◆ Sitting cross-legged on a folded blanket with the spine lifted and straight.

◆ Lying on your back on a yoga mat or a blanket on the floor in *Corpse* pose (see Chapter 7) with arms slightly away from the body and palms facing up, legs stretched straight out and relaxed. If you have a tendency to easily doze off, we recommend you do these meditations in a seated versus a supine position.

Now you are ready to meditate on your chakras. Record your voice reading each of these meditations, or ask someone to read them for you. Relax, breathe naturally, and listen, following the words and focusing your consciousness according to the directions.

Whether you or someone else reads this meditation, make sure to read it in a slow and calming manner. It can even help to make your voice almost a monotone. Also, do we have to tell you that when it says *[pause]*, you are supposed to pause but not actually say the word "pause"?

Root Chakra Meditation

Relax all the muscles in your body and soften your breath. Close your eyes. [pause]

Take a long, slow, deep inhalation. As you exhale, imagine pure energy funneling down into the base of your spine. Your first chakra begins to glow a deep ruby red, like a lustrous jewel. Your hips feel heavy, as if made from dense stone that sinks into the ground, cradled by the earth. You feel still, immovable, calm, serene, and absolutely safe. [pause]

Now, imagine you are standing at the base of a vast cliff of rock that rises high above you into the sky. The cliff face is full of deep crags and crevices, and you can barely see the top, rising into the clouds. In front of you, you see a cave, the entrance lit with candles, carpeted with soft moss; the walls are smooth and clean. Look at the entrance to this cave and contemplate what might be inside. [pause]

Step forward and enter the cave. As soon as you step inside, you see that the cavern is vast and spacious with a high vaulted ceiling. The air moves as if by a gentle breeze from somewhere, warm and comfortable. Candles flicker everywhere, casting a deep red glow over the cave's interior. The moss carpet gives way to smooth stone. Walk further into this room and look around. [pause]

Root chakra.

You notice another opening at the back of this room. It is also lit by candles that flicker warmly, so you walk into this second, smaller chamber. The room is completely empty except for the candles along the walls and a natural square-shape stone in the middle of the room. You walk over to the stone and sit on it, making yourself comfortable. You feel as if you can sit cross-legged without any effort. [pause]

As you sit, you begin to feel as if you are a part of this vast mountain. Here, inside this cave, sitting on this stone in this private room, you realize the room was designed just for you because this is your place to be safe. You feel deeply anchored to the earth as you breathe the mountain's inner air, feeling the height of the mountain above you as your own height, the cliff's crags and shelves as the vast topography of your own mind, and the mountain's weighty authority as your own inner resource, nourished and supported by the planet. [pause]

Feel your first chakra slowly spinning and strengthening, opening to the earth's reassuring body and drawing the strength of stone and mountains from its core. The ruby-red color washes over you, the candles flare with the power of the earth, and your first chakra flashes into full awareness. Inhale deeply, then exhale pure energy down your spine into your first chakra, illuminating the red wheel with sparkling light. [pause]

When you are ready, slowly rise from the stone bench, walk out of the small room, through the larger room, and back out of the cave. Look back up the cliff face and know that you are the mountain. [pause]

When you are ready, slowly move your fingers and toes and rock yourself gently back and forth. Open your eyes, and return to your day with your first chakra energized and healed.

Energy Unplugged

Whenever you need to do something that will require a certain skill or strength, do a guided meditation for the relevant chakra to help you relax beforehand. If you need to go to a job interview, visit the bank about getting a loan, or ask your boss for a raise, do a first chakra meditation. It can give you calm confidence and help you project energy that says you already have the job, the loan, or the raise.

Passion Chakra Meditation

Relax all the muscles in your body and soften your breath. Close your eyes. [pause]

Take a long, slow, deep inhalation. As you exhale, imagine pure energy funneling down into your abdomen, just behind your navel. Your second chakra begins to glow a deep fire orange, like the light from a torch. Deep inside your abdomen, you begin to feel the movement of waves, as if you contained a vast ocean inside you with a confident tide, rocking your body with its ebb and flow. [pause]

Imagine you are standing on a wide, white beach with grassy dunes behind you and an immense sea in front of you. It is dawn and the sun hasn't yet risen above the ocean, but the whole sky is colored a brilliant orange with washes of pink and textured with deep blue and purple clouds like the wisps of smoke. Watch the sky for a while. [pause]

Now, turn your gaze down to the water, which extends as far as you can see. The surf is calm and steady, with waves starting from far back and rolling gently in to break and wash calmly over the sand. Step into the water and let it surround your ankles and shins. The water is warm and swirls around you as the sky begins to brighten, the orange growing lighter and warmer and the clouds parting. The surf grows stronger and the waves pulse and flow against your knees and thighs. Feel the sea. [pause]

Passion chakra.

You move forward and dive into the water, letting the swirling warm sea caress your back and shoulders, your neck and face and hair. You come up out of the water and begin to swim, and the swimming is completely effortless. You look around, and the sea has become like a mirror. You ease onto your back and float on the quiet surface of the sea, gazing at the warm orange sky and letting the water rock you. [pause]

Feel your second chakra slowly spinning and strengthening, opening to the water's gentle pulse and flow, drawing the energy of movement and grace from the depth and breadth of the sea. The flaming orange sky washes over you and your second chakra flashes into full awareness. Inhale deeply, then exhale pure energy down your spine into your second chakra, illuminating the orange with sparkling watery light. [pause]

When you are ready, you begin swimming again, but you don't have far to go because you are almost back to shore. The sea has carried you safely to the place where you belong. Your feet find the sand and you walk out of the water as the sun rises behind you into the sky, bathing the beach, the dunes, and your body in warm light. Turn to look back at the sea, and know that you are the sea. [pause]

When you are ready, slowly move your fingers and toes and rock yourself gently back and forth. Open your eyes, and return to your day with your second chakra energized and healed.

> **Energy Unplugged**
>
> Water—the element associated with the second chakra—is a traditional symbol for passion and sexuality. Second chakra guided meditations are perfect for getting you in the mood for love, for preparing you to create something new in your life, for putting you in touch with your emotions, for balancing intense feelings, and for helping you connect more effectively with the people in your life.

Power Chakra Meditation

Relax all the muscles in your body and soften your breath. Close your eyes. [pause]

Take a long, slow, deep inhalation. As you exhale, imagine pure energy funneling down into your chest and pooling at the base of your rib cage, in your solar plexus. Your third chakra begins to glow a brilliant, dazzling gold, like the light of the sun. Deep inside your solar plexus, you begin to feel a center of warmth that spreads through your entire chest like a radiating sun. [pause]

Power chakra.

Visualize yourself standing on a tall platform in the middle of a field covered in sunflowers for as far as you can see in every direction. The huge flowers wave gently in the breeze. The sky is brilliant blue with no clouds and the sun beams down on the field with warm rays. You can feel the sun on your skin and everything looks dazzlingly beautiful—the waving acres of yellow sunflowers on thick green stalks, the bright blue sky, and the golden light. [pause]

Now, look up at the blue sky that is full of depth. You lift your arms up above your head to embrace the sun and you feel yourself rising, as if lifted by the rays, rising up off the platform and high over the field. You look down and see flowers for miles. Look up and feel the wind rushing past your face, then clouds, then nothing—you are rushing through space but always with your eye on the sun, flying like an arrow, arms outstretched. You begin to play, stretching your arms out to the side like Superman, swimming as if you were in water, turning somersaults and throwing both arms back to plunge headfirst toward the sun. Feel how fun it is to fly. [pause]

As you get closer and closer to the sun, you feel the warmth but the rays don't burn you. Instead, they feel like gentle pulsations of warmth. As you get closer, you see how huge the sun is—a massive spinning sphere of fire and lava, molten and inviting. You hold your breath, put your arms over your head, press your palms together, and dive straight into the sun, leaving ripples on the surface. Inside, you realize you are floating, suspended, in the middle of the sun, supported by light and fire. You see Earth, far away, green and blue, spinning around you. You smile as you realize that suddenly, just for a few glorious moments, the earth really does revolve around you! [pause]

Feel your third chakra slowly spinning and strengthening, opening to the sun's power and rays of light as it flashes into full awareness, light pouring out of your solar plexus in rays that reach far beyond you, merging and becoming the light of the sun. Inhale deeply, then exhale pure energy down your spine into your third chakra, setting the gold aglow with sparkling rays of light. [pause]

When you are ready, relax into the sun's warmth and begin to float down, slowly, then pick up speed, not falling but flying, back toward Earth and back to the field of sunflowers where you land gently back on the platform. You turn your face back up to the sun, and know that you are the sun. [pause]

When you are ready, slowly move your fingers and toes and rock yourself gently back and forth. Open your eyes, and return to your day with your third chakra energized and healed.

> **Energy Unplugged**
>
> Our entire world exists because of the sun. When you envision the sun inside you, it can infuse you with great personal power, but tempered by warmth and charisma.

Heart Chakra Meditation

Relax all the muscles in your body and soften your breath. Close your eyes. [pause]

Take a long, slow, deep inhalation. As you exhale, imagine pure energy filling up your heart. Your fourth chakra begins to glow bright emerald green, like a glowing jewel. Deep inside your heart, you begin to feel a flowering, as if your heart were filled with vines and leaves and buds slowly unfolding and gently blossoming. [pause]

Heart chakra.

Imagine you are standing at the base of a huge leafy tree with a thick knotty trunk and hundreds of magnificent sturdy branches lushly covered in brilliant green leaves. You look up through the branches and see layers of leaves and twigs. Feel the roots under your feet and look up at the branches extending into the sky. Reach out and grab hold of the thick sturdy bark and begin to climb. [pause]

It feels good to pull yourself up the tree. Whenever you need a branch to hold or a knot to stand on, there it is. You climb easily and freely, higher and higher until you can't see the ground anymore. Still you climb higher until the branches begin to thin and you realize you are almost at the top. You can see light above you now so you climb faster. At the very top of the tree, you find a seat in a wide V-shaped branch. You can see for miles and miles—fields, mountains, forests, and blue sky. [pause]

A gentle wind rises and the tree begins to sway back and forth, rocking you like a swing. At the tip of each branch, tiny buds burst into more leaves, filling up all the spaces beneath you so you feel completely secure and nurtured by this wise and sentient tree. The leaves brush against you, making gentle whispering sounds. [pause]

Feel your fourth chakra slowly spinning and strengthening, opening to the green leaves and powerful branches. The tree glows with a green light and your heart feels as if it were a bud bursting open with leaves, flashing into full awareness. Green light pours from your heart, filling up your chest and flowing into your shoulders and arms and out your fingertips. Inhale deeply, then exhale pure energy into your fourth chakra, illuminating it with sparkling, leafy-green light. [pause]

When you are ready, begin your descent, climbing easily back down the tree, through the branches and leaves that move to support and care for you. You feel deeply loved and nurtured. Finally you reach the ground. Look up, your gaze following the sturdy trunk up into the branches and leaves of the magnificent tree, and know that you are the tree. [pause]

When you are ready, slowly move your fingers and toes and rock yourself gently back and forth. Open your eyes, and return to your day with your fourth chakra energized and healed.

> **Energy Unplugged**
>
> Heart chakra meditations are perfect when you are having trouble feeling compassion toward someone—including yourself.

Throat Chakra Meditation

Relax all the muscles in your body and soften your breath. Close your eyes. [pause]

Take a long, slow, deep inhalation. As you exhale, imagine pure energy rising up into your throat. Your fifth chakra begins to glow bright sapphire blue, like a brilliant jewel. Deep inside your throat, you feel a gentle, subtle vibration that slowly grows and grows until you realize music lives inside you. [pause]

Imagine you are walking through the woods on a path covered in pine needles. Trees surround you on either side and sunlight pours through between the branches. Among the trees, deer watch you. Birds flutter back and forth between the branches. A fox darts inside a hollow log to your right, and you catch just a glimpse of his big fluffy tail. A stream runs along beside the path, and as you walk, you pass a raccoon dipping his paws into the water. Everywhere you look, you see animals and you know this is their home, but you are welcome here. [pause]

Truth chakra.

You come upon a large log between the path and the stream. It looks comfortable, so you sit and settle in where a thick branch makes a perfect rest for your back. Lean into the log, relax, and listen. [pause]

The first thing you hear is all the different birds singing, and the way all their songs weave into one another like a chorus of voices. Then you hear the gentle background sound of the stream pouring over rocks as it moves through the woods. The wind in the pine trees adds another layer of sound ... the pattering rustle of poplar trees and the soft swishing sound of oak trees. Then you hear finer sounds: the air, the sun hitting the forest floor, the light and clouds and space, the planet spinning and the solar system turning like a giant chakra. Everything makes a sound and all the sounds harmonize into one beautiful song. [pause]

Feel your fifth chakra spinning and strengthening, opening to the song of the earth and sky and the sound of being. The forest glows with blue light as it sings and your fifth chakra flashes into full awareness. Inhale deeply, then exhale pure energy into your fifth chakra, illuminating it with sparkling blue, sound-drenched light. [pause]

When you are ready, take a deep breath, then rise from the log and walk back down the path, past the raccoon, squirrels, and deer. As you leave the woods, you turn and look and know that you are the singing woods. [pause]

When you are ready, slowly move your fingers and toes and rock yourself gently back and forth. Open your eyes, and return to your day with your fifth chakra energized and healed.

Energy Unplugged _____

If you are struggling with telling someone your real feelings, or you can't quite get the words out, try a fifth chakra meditation. This chakra puts you in touch with your ability to listen to others, as well as speak your truth in an honest and forthright way.

Third Eye Chakra Meditation

Relax all the muscles in your body and soften your breath. Close your eyes. [pause]

Take a long, slow, deep inhalation. As you exhale, imagine pure energy rising up into your forehead and pooling at your third eye, just above the space between your eyebrows. Your sixth chakra begins to glow a deep indigo-purple, like a dark amethyst with an inner glow that illuminates your mind with a wash of gentle violet light, like the sky at dusk. [pause]

Third Eye chakra.

Imagine that you have a room inside your head, and the door is in your third eye, just above the space between your eyebrows. Whenever you want to go inside yourself to think, figure out what to do about something, contemplate your beliefs, or just get away from it all, you can go into this room, close the door, and have time completely to yourself. Visualize stepping into this room and closing the door behind you. Look around the room. It can be any shape, any size, any color, any style you want. What will you make of it? Does it have windows? Carpet or wood floor? What color are the walls? Anything you envision for the room happens before your eyes. Create your room now. [pause]

You can furnish the room with anything you like. Do you want a luxurious bed in the corner? A fireplace, fountain, pool, or steamy hot tub? Do you want a desk, table, magnificent kitchen, cushioned window seat? Chandeliers? Candles? Walls of books? An easel? A meditation garden? Your room may be full or almost empty. If you add something and you don't like it, you can make it disappear again. Move things around until you get the room exactly the way you want it. Don't worry about making permanent decisions, either. The next time you come to your room, you can change it around completely. How will your room look today? Furnish your room now. [pause]

Find a comfortable spot in your room to sit and get comfortable. Let your mind open to what you need right now. Why do you need time alone right now? What are you looking for? What answers do you seek? [pause]

As you sit in quiet contemplation, feel your sixth chakra slowly spinning and strengthening, opening to the inner turning that is yours in this room. See the room growing lighter until your sixth chakra flashes into full awareness. Inhale deeply, then exhale pure energy into your sixth chakra, illuminating it with sparkling violet light. [pause]

Energy Unplugged

You are more than your thoughts, but sometimes we all need to get better control over our thoughts and steady them in order to move forward in our lives. This is the time for sixth chakra meditation, for it helps us tap into our deep inner wisdom that has all the answers we ever need.

When you are ready, take a deep breath, stand, walk to the door, open it, then turn back to see your beautiful room and know that the room in your mind is your mind, and you can make it into anything you need. [pause]

When you are ready, slowly move your fingers and toes and rock yourself gently back and forth. Open your eyes, and return to your day with your sixth chakra energized and healed.

Crown Chakra Meditation

Relax all the muscles in your body and soften your breath. Close your eyes. [pause]

Take a long, slow, deep inhalation. As you exhale, imagine pure energy rising up into the crown of your head and pooling at your seventh chakra, which begins to glow like a sparkling diamond rotating slowly about an inch above the crown of your head. As you focus on this brilliant jewel, it begins to change, unfolding into a beautiful white lotus flower with one thousand petals. [pause]

Thousand-Petaled Lotus chakra.

You are piloting a small ship through space. Although you've never been trained to do it, you already know exactly how to operate the controls and you fly easily past thousands of stars and spinning planets. Your ship has windows on every side and as you fly, easily avoiding any collisions, you can see the velvety blackness of space and the brilliant luminous objects all around you—clouds of dust that seem to be lit from within, lazy meteors and soaring comets with long glowing tails. Far off in the distance, you see a glow brighter and more incandescent than all the other dazzling stars and planets. It looks like a giant star. You turn your ship to fly toward it and as you get closer, you see it is a solid sphere, not a star, with a stable surface that radiates an inner light. You land, step out of your ship, and know you will be able to breathe. As your feet touch the ground, you begin to glow, illuminated by the surface. Begin to explore, infused with a quiet calm; as you walk, the surface undulates and glows, changing shapes, rising up into waves or forms like pillars or spheres, then sinking back into itself so that the landscape you walk over is in constant flux. Yet your footing is never unsure. Every shape looks familiar. Stop and watch the surface of this glowing landscape shifting. [pause]

You hear a low humming wind whispering a message directly into your mind: You are this. As you listen and try to understand, you feel your seventh chakra slowly spinning and strengthening and the thousand-petaled lotus that is your Crown chakra begins to open, petal by petal, blossoming into a giant rotating flower above your head.

Suddenly you understand that just when you have reached the threshold of finally comprehending what life is, there will always be more, a never-ending unfolding. Your seventh chakra flashes into full awareness and suddenly you understand that it is all one—you, the planet, stars, meteors and comets, earth, clouds, sky, sea, forests and trees, mountains and cliffs. It is all you, and you are a part of all, rising up like a wave then falling back into universal consciousness. Inhale deeply, then exhale pure energy into your seventh chakra, illuminating it with sparkling diamond light. [pause]

When you are ready, take a deep breath, then walk back to your ship, climb inside, close the door, and rise back up off this strange yet familiar planet. As you lift off, turn back to see the glowing surface, and know that you are the glowing surface, and that when you return to Earth, you will be Earth, too, and everything in it will be you. [pause]

When you are ready, slowly move your fingers and toes and rock yourself gently back and forth. Open your eyes, and return to your day with your seventh chakra energized and healed.

The Least You Need to Know

- Guided chakra meditation is a good way to learn about meditation because it is easier to focus on a voice leading you through visualization than to just sit and clear your mind.

- To practice chakra meditation, find a comfortable, clean place where you won't be interrupted. Either record yourself reading the guided meditation, or ask someone to read it for you while you meditate.

- Guided meditations for each chakra use symbolism and imagery associated with that chakra to help energize and balance the chakra.

Part 5

Relax, Release, Restore, Renew

In this final part of the book, you learn even more advanced ways of working with your chakras. The part starts with a chapter on how to go even further finding and releasing blockages in your chakras, using yoga poses and other basic physical movements. We move on to show you how visualization can be a powerful tool for chakra healing and maintenance, and then we get super spiritual with a lesson on your very own astral and causal bodies.

JUST SO YOU KNOW, I'VE DISCOVERED THAT MY ASTRAL BODY IS *WAY* HOTTER THAN MY PHYSICAL ONE!

BARR

Chapter 18

The Power of Two: Partner Work for Releasing Blocks and Balancing Overloads

In This Chapter

- Why two chakras are sometimes better than one
- How chakras equalize
- Yin, yang, and chakras
- Partner exercise for balancing the chakras

"People … people who need people … are the luckiest peeee-pllllle, in the wooooorld …." Okay, we'll stop. We realize you really don't want to hear us do karaoke versions of 1960s hits. However, we dabble in song just to make a point: chakras seek each other.

In fact, chakra magnetism is one of the coolest things about chakras, and we have a theory about it. We think that maybe the reason humans are such social animals, always seeking companionship—friends as well as sexual partners and soul mates—is because our chakras are drawn to the chakras of other people. Maybe that's one of our primary connections.

In the same way that making a particular sound can tone and tune up the chakras (see Chapter 15), so can close contact with the chakra of another. The best thing about synchronizing your chakras with someone else's chakras is that chakras don't synchronize their blocks or overloads. The healthiest, most balanced chakra opens or balances the less balanced chakra, and if you and a partner have different chakra strengths, each one's strength will benefit the other, without any negative effects from unbalanced chakras. In other words, only good can come of chakra partner work!

That's what this chapter is about. We show you how to tune up your chakras with some simple exercises with another person. This can be your partner, your soul mate, or your friend. You can even do these exercises with your children, although they work best if you are approximately the same size, so your chakras line up.

First, let's talk about why chakra synchronizing works.

Chakra Synchronicity

If you hold a pendulum over a chakra, the energy or *prana* in that chakra will rise up toward the pendulum like a bubble seeking the surface of the water, or a piece of iron drawn to a magnet. like a portal.

That's because *prana* tends to seek other *prana*. You can actually feel this magnetic like attraction. Rub your two palms together briskly until they begin to feel warm. Then, close your eyes (so you aren't distracted by visual stimulus) and put your palms close together but not quite touching. Move them slowly wider apart, then closer together. Pay close attention to the feeling in your palms. Can you feel the energy buzzing and flowing, one palm to the other? Can you feel it pulling as you pull your palms apart, as if it wants you to bring your palms together?

Spinning Your Wheels _____

We believe our chakras are attracted to the chakras of other people, and we also believe our chakras are attracted to the chakras of animals. Yes, animals have chakras, too, that can open and close, get blocked or overloaded, much the same as we do. In an animal, the Root chakra lies at the base of the tail, the Passion chakra in the lower abdomen, the Solar Plexus chakra at the base of the rib cage, the Heart chakra at the heart, the Throat chakra in the throat, the Third Eye chakra at the forehead, and the Crown chakra at the highest point of the skull. Perhaps that's why people are so fascinated with animals, and why we have developed such close and meaningful relationships with our dogs and cats.

That's because you have small chakras in both your palms, and they seek each other's energy. Maybe that's why it feels so good to hold someone's hand. Your hand chakras are communing.

The Yin-Yang Connection

Chakras also attract each other because of yin and yang. In case you don't remember the yin-yang discussion in Chapter 3, the concept of yin and yang comes from China and says that yin and yang are opposite but balancing forces inherent in everything. Yin is the lunar, feminine, cooling, receptive, earthy, wild, undisciplined energy. It is also the energy of *Kudalini*. Yang is the solar, masculine, heating, forceful, disciplined, structured, spiritual energy, and the masculine counterpart to *Kundalini*, which is Shiva in Indian philosophy. Yin urges yang into a more sensual and joyful appreciation of life, while yang urges yin into a more evolved spiritual understanding of existence.

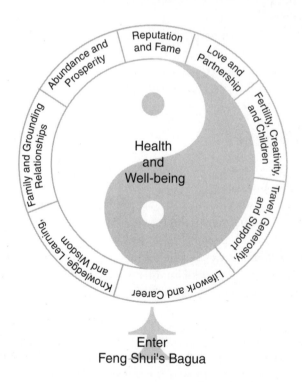

Yin and yang also influence the Eastern practice of Feng shui, which studies the flow of energy through personal spaces. Think of the areas in Feng Shui's bagua (like an energy map) as the chakras of your house!

The yin-yang symbol is a circle that is half black and half white, with a swirl of each fitting inside the other, and a dot of the opposite color inside each swirl. It represents ultimate balance. You have both yin and yang energy in you and every one of your chakras has yin and yang energy spinning inside it.

According to the Chinese, all things seek to balance their yin and yang. You can apply this to the chakras in different ways, but let's take the Heart chakra as an example. When your Heart chakra is blocked and you have a hard time giving and receiving love, you may have too much yang, which is more intellectual and spiritual and less immersed in communion with the physical world. If, on the other hand, you give love too easily with wild abandon and don't logically consider the consequences of being too open or letting others manipulate you because you love them so much, you may have too much yin.

But put an overloaded Heart chakra or a blocked Heart chakra right up against a healthy, balanced Heart chakra that processes energy according to its nature, and the blocks can melt, the overloads even out. The two Heart chakras synchronize, always balancing out according to the healthiest chakra.

Another way to look at it is that the energy or *prana* within your chakras is like water that always seeks to rejoin the sea. All chakras—indeed, all bodies—have within them an innate sense of what it feels like to be open and healthy, because an open, healthy chakra has direct access to universal *prana* that flows in and out of it. The sea doesn't seek to flow up into the rivers and dams and lakes, and universal *prana* doesn't align itself with blocks or overloads. Instead, when a troubled chakra detects a healthy chakra, it tends to align itself with that chakra because it recognizes its true nature.

Chakra Partner Exercise

This tendency of the chakras to seek and balance each other makes partner work a natural way to clear blocks and balance overloads in your own chakras. This kind of work can be as simple as a hug. When you hug someone, many of your primary chakras are put into direct contact with each other—especially at the chest, heart, and throat. That feels good, and that's probably part of why hugs have been proven to be physically and psychologically beneficial. The strongest of each of the chakras helps open the weaker of the chakras, getting them all spinning and active again. Hugs are particularly beneficial for opening the Heart chakra. (See the "Heart to Heart" exercise later in this chapter.)

But you and your partner, friend, or family member can help each other even more, with targeted chakra partner work. As long as you choose someone you trust, these exercises can really make an impact on your own chakras. Plus, partner work is mutually beneficial, so your strongest chakras can make a big impact on your partner, too.

Energy Unplugged

Making love is the ultimate chakra partner exercise. When you make love with your partner, you are not only aligning your Heart chakras, but you are also aligning your Root, Passion, and Power chakras—all the earthy chakras that ground you and give you access to an appreciation of the physical world. When you kiss, you are aligning your Throat and Third Eye chakras, too. Yes, a really good kiss can stimulate your natural intuition and sense of what is right.

Meditation: Back-to-Back

We usually think of the chakras from the front of the body, but they are actually inside the body, in the middle, and their energy emanates out of the back of the body, too. However, the fronts of our bodies represent our vulnerable, personal selves (the yin side of the body), while the backs of our bodies represent our more detached, universal, spiritual selves (the yang side of the body).

For this reason, back-to-back partner work is a great place to begin. Both partners won't feel quite as vulnerable or nervous if they line up their universal sides, as opposed to their personal sides. Sitting back-to-back is also an excellent way to meditate in synch. You just focus on meditating, and each partner's spiritual nature will become ignited by the close contact of your spiritual sides and the alignment of your chakras, making meditation easier and more effective.

You can meditate back-to-back with a partner any time, but in this exercise, meditation is a preparation for other, more personal chakra work because it increases each partner's immediate awareness of his or her chakras. You don't have to think about the other person's chakras at all, and even though you aren't doing anything purposefully, your chakras will be aligning and strengthening each other, just because of their close contact.

As for what *you* have to do with conscious intention, just think of this exercise as tuning in to your chakra channels so you can get the station to come in without any static. Then you can listen to the music.

1. Position a folded blanket on the floor or in the middle of a yoga mat. Sit back-to-back with your partner, so that each of you is sitting on the opposite edge of the blanket. Your lower backs should be touching and you can rest against each other a little, so that as much of your backs come together as possible without one person pushing harder on the other. You should both be sitting up straight.

2. Imagine you are both rising up from the crown of the head to straighten your spines. Breathe naturally and listen to your breath. Don't worry about how your partner is breathing, although you may find that your breath naturally begins to synchronize with your partner's breath, without any effort. Just keep focusing on your own breath. This is the time to center your mind on you and your own chakras, so you are in the right mode to do more with them in subsequent exercises. If you need to readjust or have any concerns, just say so. It is perfectly okay for you to talk, or laugh for that matter.

3. Now it's time to tune in to your chakras. You each have a job to do. You are going to take turns naming the chakras, and as you do, both partners focus all their attention on their own named chakra. Choose who will go first.

4. The first partner says: *Root.* Bring all your attention to your own Root chakra. Don't worry about feeling your partner's chakra right now. You are back-to-back, so that part will take care of itself. Just think about your own. Feel your Root chakra spinning at the base of your spine. Imagine its red color and its power to ground you. Breathe normally and feel your chakra for about 30 seconds. It's okay to look at a clock or watch while you do this.

5. The second partner says: *Passion.* Bring all your attention to your own Passion chakra and feel it spinning just below your navel. Imagine its orange color and feel its power to move you and inspire your emotions and creativity. Focus on this chakra for about 30 seconds, breathing normally.

6. The first partner says: *Power.* Bring all your attention to your Power chakra and feel it spinning at the base of your rib cage, at your solar plexus. Imagine its yellow color and feel how it projects your own personal power and confidence, giving you the will to act, change, and make things happen. Focus on this chakra for about 30 seconds, breathing normally.

7. The second partner says: *Heart.* Bring all your attention to your Heart chakra and feel it spinning around your heart, in the center of your chest. Imagine its green color and feel how it infuses your entire torso with compassion, love, and healing energy. Focus on this chakra for about 30 seconds, breathing normally.

8. The first partner says: *Throat.* Bring all your attention to your Throat chakra and feel it spinning in your throat, right behind the hollow between your collarbones. Imagine its blue color and feel how it ignites your inner sense of perception, discerning the truth of situations and being able to speak and listen with intelligence and clarity. Focus on this chakra for about 30 seconds, breathing normally.

9. The second partner says: *Third Eye.* Bring all your attention to your Third Eye chakra and feel it spinning in your forehead, just above the space between your eyebrows. Imagine its deep indigo color and feel how it activates your intuition so that you know much more than you can perceive with your five senses. Your inner knowing glows. Focus on this chakra for about 30 seconds, breathing normally.

10. The first partner says: *Crown.* Bring all your attention to your Crown chakra and feel it spinning just above the crown of your head. Imagine its pure purple or pure white color and feel how it opens to a universal sense of knowledge, power, and spirit that is beyond you and yet within you, connecting you to everything. Focus on this chakra for about 30 seconds breathing normally.

11. The second partner says: *Return.* Breathe deeply and bring your awareness back to the external world. Feel your partner's back against yours. Both partners rock back and forth gently to re-energize their legs. Slowly lean forward and come back up to standing. Face your partner, bring your palms together in front of your heart, and say *thank you.*

Now you are ready to do more.

Energy Unplugged

Having a clear, conscious intention is one of the most important things you can do to increase the effectiveness of any chakra work. Before you begin any chakra exercise, always set your intention. What do you want to happen? Just think about the answer for a moment, or fill in the blank to this sentence: *Right now, I do this because* _____. Your answers will vary, but might be something like *because I want to open my heart*, or *because I want to feel more confident in who I am*, or *because I want to say what I really mean*. Setting your intention isn't just good for chakra work. It is good to do before you attempt anything, whether you are working on a project for your job (*because I am committed to fulfilling my role in the team*), taking a yoga class (*because I want to feel stronger and more flexible today*), or just getting ready to cook dinner (*because I want to nourish myself with good food*).

Chakra Line-Up: Palm-to-Palm

This exercise is excellent for romantic partners because it really brings two people closer together and can generate strong feelings of compassion and even desire. However, this is not a sexual exercise, it is an intimacy exercise.

This exercise is designed to help increase your feelings of integration as a couple, but it also works very well for two friends who are not romantically involved, helping them to forge a deeper and more meaningful connection. It is also incredibly healing because throughout the exercise, you join palms with your partner, so the healing energy that flows from your Heart chakras out through your palms is twice as strong, as it mingles with your partner's healing energy.

This exercise is also ideal for aligning and balancing all the chakras—yours and your partner's—because you work through each chakra, as you did in the first exercise. In this one, however, since you are face-to-face, focusing on the more vulnerable and personal side of your body and consciously connecting your chakras, the impact of the partnership is more intense and powerful.

Before you begin, decide who will start when cueing each chakra. If you just finished the previous exercise, switch who goes first. Spend about 30 seconds on each chakra, but if you know one or both of you is having issues with a particular chakra, allow a little more time with that chakra—up to one minute.

1. Stand in Mountain pose (see Chapter 7), about two feet from your partner, face-to-face. Both partners stand with their feet shoulder-width apart. Arms hang at your sides. Stand up straight, lengthen the sides of your body as you pull your shoulders up, then roll them back, opening your chest. Move your upper inner thighs apart and back, and keep your tailbone tucked under. Keep a very slight bend in your knees. Stand comfortably and breathe normally.

2. Both partners hold out their arms and grasp each other's wrists with straight arms. Bend your knees and stick your buttocks way back as you pull against each other, like you are water-skiing. You may need to take a step back to find the correct balance. Keeping your arms straight, stretch your arms and shoulders while keeping your armpits lifting. Get in synch with each other's energy.

3. Stand, release wrists, step closer to your partner, and then hold out your hands at the level of your Heart chakra, palms facing your partner. Touch your palms to the palms of your partner.

4. Close your eyes, keeping your palms together. The first partner says: *One.* Both partners focus all their attention on the energy of their first chakras. Imagine your first chakra's deep red color and vigorous spin at the base of your spine, and then imagine it moving outward like a funnel to join the energy of your partner's first chakra. You are rooted together like a great double-trunked tree. Visualize each chakra growing and strengthening, opening fully and coming in line with

its fellow chakra. Both chakras fill up with energy and powerful red light. Keep the connection between your palms.

5. After about 30 seconds, the second partner says: *Two.* Both partners focus all their attention on the energy of their second chakras. Imagine your second chakra's fiery orange color and flowing, undulating spin in your lower abdomen, and then imagine it moving outward like a funnel to join the energy of your partner's second chakra. You are joined by your emotions. Visualize each chakra growing and strengthening, opening fully and coming in line with its fellow chakra. Both chakras fill up with energy and fiery orange light. Keep the connection between your palms and all your lower chakras.

6. After about 30 seconds, the first partner says: *Three.* Repeat the process for the remaining chakras. For each chakra, both partners focus all their attention on the energy of that chakra, imagining the color (yellow for the third, green for the fourth, blue for the fifth, indigo for the sixth, purple or white for the seventh) and the chakra's energetic spin, then imagine it moving outward like a funnel to join the energy of your partner's corresponding chakra, connecting you. For each chakra, visualize your joined chakras growing and strengthening, opening fully and coming in line with its fellow. Throughout the exercise, keep the connection between your palms and all your lower chakras.

7. After about 30 seconds, the second partner says: After you have finished the seventh chakra, open your eyes. Put your palms together in front of your Heart chakra and thank your partner.

> **Energy Unplugged**
>
> Chakra partner work should be fun and lighthearted because if one person begins to feel intimidated or manipulated, their chakras might close reactively. Laugh, smile, be supportive of each other, and have a good time. The more open you are, the more open your chakras will be.

A Hug a Day: Heart-to-Heart

Is a hug a day good medicine? You bet it is, because when you hug someone, your Heart chakras touch and they get a chance to fortify and strengthen each other. Because the Heart chakra is the source of healing energy in the body's energy system, hugs are particularly alchemical.

When two Heart chakras physically make contact, the combined energy becomes greater than the sum of its parts and infuses both partners with a real feeling of well-being and increased inner healing.

1. Find a willing partner, of any size. Kids are great. Open your arms.

2. Instead of putting your right arm up over your partner's shoulder and your left arm under their right arm (the typical hug move), go the other way: your left arm over their shoulder and your right arm under their left arm. This puts your actual hearts closer together.

3. Squeeze and hold for at least 10 seconds. Don't worry about what your Heart chakra is doing because it knows exactly how to heal. Work up to 30 second hugs.

4. Repeat several times daily.

Hugging seems simple, even a formality, but regular Heart chakra bonding with other human beings not only makes you feel better but increases your sense of connectedness with all life. When you feel connected, you feel happier, calmer, and more satisfied with your life. Studies also suggest that regular hugs actually boost your immune function. We suggest you work up to 10 of them a day, if possible.

Spinning Your Wheels

According to a study conducted at the University of North Carolina, hugs increase the body's production of oxytocin, which is the chemical that makes you feel emotionally connected to and nurturing toward other people. According to the study, when two people hugged for 20 seconds, oxytocin levels increased, especially between people who already loved each other. Oxytocin doesn't just make you feel nurturing toward someone. It has also been shown to reduce the risk of heart disease. At the same time, levels of cortisol—the notorious "stress hormone"—decreased during the 20-second hug. Cortisol has also been linked to heart disease. Is it a coincidence that touching Heart chakras decreases the risk of heart disease? We don't think so.

Seeing Clearly: Third Eye-to-Third Eye

The sensitive Third Eye chakra is particularly susceptible to the energy of others, so even though this is a quick exercise, it packs a punch. Don't be alarmed if you "see" visions or images during this exercise. Opening your Intuition chakra so close to someone else's can cause this to happen. If you want this to happen, stay very calm, breathe deeply, and really concentrate on opening your Third Eye chakra like a window.

Take turns exploring your Heart chakras by sharing forward and backward bends. How open is your heart to your partner? This pose can be seen as a metaphor for the yin and yang balance of partnership through the Heart chakra.

You may see symbolic images or events related to yourself or to your partner during this exercise. If you do, talk about it with your partner to figure out if what you see means something to either one or both of you. If you don't see anything, that's okay, too. Intuition comes in many forms, and it isn't always trying to tell you something. Even when your intuition is silent, this exercise is healthful and strengthening to your sixth chakra.

1. Stand face-to-face with your partner, about six inches apart, in Mountain pose (see Chapter 7), with your feet a little less than shoulder-width apart, your arms at your sides, and your back straight.

2. Look your partner in the eye and begin breathing together to a count of approximately five seconds inhaling, five seconds exhaling. With each inhalation, imagine the crown of your head rising, to expand and make space inside your body. With each exhalation, imagine your body expanding, so that your energy reaches out in every direction.

3. Keep breathing together. Slowly, so you don't bump heads, both partners lean in toward each other and touch foreheads. Synchronize your breathing by tuning in to the sound of your breath and your partner's breath You can close your eyes.

4. Stand with your foreheads touching for 10 breaths. An inhalation and an exhalation is one breath. After the tenth breath, slowly separate and stand up again.

Share with each other what you felt. You can do this again a few times, if you felt you were on the verge of seeing or feeling something and you want to give the exercise more time to work.

> **¡!!) Wake-Up Call** _____
>
> Touching your Third Eye to someone else's Third Eye is a powerful exercise, so don't overdo it. You should not hold this pose for more than 20 breaths unless you both have a lot of practice meditating and are both comfortable with it. Otherwise, the physical posture can strain your back, and the intense electrical energy through your Third Eye chakra could cause a chakra imbalance, opening your Third Eye chakra too much, at the expense of your other chakras.

Open your chakras side-by-side with yoga's Tree pose. Hold each other's feet and rest your opposite hands on the small of your backs. As you stand your ground together, feel your chakras opening and spreading like branches of two trees growing and intertwining their energy.

Savasana: Crown-to-Crown

In this easy but enlightening exercise, you and a partner lie in the classic yoga pose called *Savasana* or Corpse pose (Chapter 7), but you lie with the crowns of your heads touching, or very close together. This joining of Crown chakras magnifies the energy in each person's Crown chakra, attracting more external *prana* to flow into all your chakras and encouraging all your internal *prana* to flow upward. You may feel a strong sense of connectedness to all life and a deep sense of well-being during and/or after this exercise. You may also feel more oriented toward your spiritual side.

Before you begin, set a timer for 10 or 15 minutes.

1. Position two yoga mats or blankets on the floor, end to end. Each partner sits in the middle of the mat, back to back with the other partner. Lie down slowly, being careful not to knock heads, and adjust so that the crowns of your heads are touching.

2. Shift your shoulder blades back under you so your chest lifts and your shoulder blades feel like they are cradling your heart. Relax your low back and slightly tuck your tailbone. Feel your neck and shoulders release.

3. Close your eyes. Relax your jaw, your teeth, your tongue. Let your eyes sink and relax the inner corners of your eyes. Relax your ears, your neck, your shoulders, your chest. Relax your arms, elbows, wrists, and hands. Relax your stomach, abdomen, hips, legs, knees, ankles, and feet. Let your entire body sink into the ground. If you lose direct contact with your partner's head, that's okay. Your seventh chakras are already joined.

4. Remain in a totally relaxed position and focus on the sound of your breath, letting your mind relax. When thoughts come to you, let them go. Thoughts will continue to arise, so acknowledge them without judgment, then let them float away. Stay in this position for about 10 minutes. You don't have to think about, visualize, or do anything about your seventh chakra during this exercise. It is an open portal to universal life force energy that flows in through you, through your partner, back out, and in through your partner, through you, and back out, in a great circle (like a giant chakra or spiral galaxy) that grows stronger and brighter with every breath.

5. When the time is up, very slowly move your fingers and toes to reorient yourself to the physical world. Slowly bend your knees and roll over to your right side. When you are ready, slowly sit up, put your palms together in front of your heart, rest a moment, then thank your partner.

 Wake-Up Call _____

If the crown-to-crown seventh chakra exercise becomes too intense, do something grounding afterward, like eating something or exercising your body.

If you don't have anyone at home who you can do this with, enlist an interested friend, or even someone from your yoga class. Show them this book and tell them what you'd like to try. When the right partner comes along for this kind of work, you'll know it.

The Least You Need to Know

- Working with a partner to open, energize, and balance your chakras is a powerful and effective tool.

- When two chakras synchronize, the healthier, more open chakra tends to "fix" the blocked or overloaded chakra, bringing it back into balance. Blocked or overloaded chakras can't negatively affect healthy, open chakras.

- Touching chakras together, such as hugging to join two Heart chakras, energizes and balances them, but you can also stand close to a partner and visualize the energy of your chakras joining.

Chapter

19

Chakra Visualizations

In This Chapter

◆ Can you really see your own chakras?

◆ The difference between imagination and perception

◆ Visualization techniques for seeing your own chakras *right now*

◆ Honing your skill

Some people come into this world automatically able to see chakras—not just their own, but everybody else's, too. Even as kids, they go through life wondering what those colored lights on everybody's bodies are, or they just accept that everyone has them and don't think to question it.

For most of us, however, seeing one's own chakras seems a little bit like seeing one's own soul. We may not really believe we can see them because they don't have a physical form. Seeing mysterious energy centers in our bodies seems a little incredible—more like something we could imagine happening than something that we believe could really happen.

But it can happen. Regular seeing is one of our physical senses, which is the realm of the three lower chakras. Seeing chakras is a more advanced skill than regular seeing because it is based on finely tuned intuition, which requires more mature development in our three upper chakras, something that takes a little more work.

Seeing Is Believing

You could read this book from the beginning all the way up to this point and still not totally believe that chakras are a real thing. That's because the concept of chakras and their symbolism are such useful tools for explaining and understanding the human psyche.

Even if we see the chakra system as one giant psychological metaphor, chakras make sense and are rewarding to explore. You might be thinking, "Yes, I have trouble opening up to love, so my Heart chakra is 'blocked,'" as in, "The *idea* of a blocked Heart chakra *symbolizes* my problems opening up to love. That makes sense to me, so now maybe I can do something about it."

That's all fine and good. In fact, it's a little like doing yoga for exercise rather than for spiritual enlightenment. It works, it's certainly not harmful, and it's fun. It makes you feel good, so you do it, even if it doesn't mean the same thing to you as it does to someone who follows the yoga path—all of it, not just the poses—in order to become enlightened.

However, once you start to *see* your chakras, you might be ready to take this whole chakra thing (and this whole yoga thing, for that matter) to the next level. Seeing your chakras, although certainly not an infallible proof of their existence (our senses can play tricks on us), can certainly make them more real to you, especially when what you see makes perfect sense with how you feel and how your life works.

A quick way to visualize your chakras open and aligned is by practicing yoga's Prana Arch pose. You can practice this pose anywhere, anytime. In the illustration, you can see how the Heart and Throat chakras are energized as your posture improves and your palms open, fingertips stretching toward the floor.

Imagination vs. Perception

When working on chakra visualization, a lot of people ask (and many more probably wonder silently) something along the lines of: "How do I know I'm not just imagining this?" Imagination can be vivid, so it's perfectly natural to wonder whether your chakra perceptions are valid or not.

Because the chakras are not physical structure, the line can get blurry, especially because the imagination is a tool for developing visualization skill. However, imagination can get in the way of intuition, like the person who is always sure she shouldn't get on that plane because she *just has a feeling it is going to crash*, when in reality, her imagination is just being fueled by anxiety about the flight or the trip itself or anything else.

But intuition is the key to telling the difference between imagination and perception. When you can calm the mind's chatter through the practice of meditation (via learning how to withdraw the senses and concentrate on a single point, eventually training the mind to quiet), that is when intuition's messages come through.

The only way to do *that* is to practice, practice, practice. Meditate on a regular basis and train your mind to see beyond the part of it that thinks, to the vast being beyond thought. Esoteric? You bet, but it works, and it's a practice worth doing if you want to really tell the difference between what your mind thinks and what your mind *knows*.

However, we aren't going to keep you in suspense. We aren't going to require you to meditate every day for an hour for the next decade before we tell you how to see your own chakras. Just know that the more you meditate and the more you learn to still your mind, the more you will be able to do the exercises in this chapter with confidence that you are authentically sensing and seeing your chakras.

There is an old Zen saying about seeing the moon's reflection in a pond. If the surface of the pond is agitated and full of ripples, the moon's reflection won't look anything like the moon. That agitation, those ripples, are your constant thoughts and feelings, which disturb your ability to perceive truth. When the pond is perfectly still, however—when your thoughts and feelings withdraw and stay quiet—then you can see the moon's reflection. You can perceive the truth. And you can see your chakras.

However, you can still see a scattered, fragmented reflection in an agitated pond. You can look as you work on calming the waters. This kind of work may even inspire you to meditate more. So let's give it a try.

Chakra Survey

You could go to a mirror and look long and hard at your body, and if you are like a few gifted people, you might be able to begin to perceive your chakras. But again, most of us need more help than that. Although chakra seeing is different from imagining, it can start with imagining, via visualization.

Visualization uses the imagination as a structure to help the mind perceive what is really going on. It can be a highly effective tool to plumb the depths of the subconscious where much of our knowing and the source of our intuition lives. This is also the source of our knowing whether our chakra visualization is accurate.

When you get more experienced, you can look at all your chakras in one session, but to get started, it's a good idea to work on them one at a time. You will have time to perceive more, instead of being tempted to rush through. Do one a day, or do them one after the other for as long as you can pay attention. Let's start with your first chakra. Are you ready to take a look?

As with other visualizations in this book, you can record yourself or someone else reading these exercises. Or read them over a few times before you do them, and if you think you remember well enough, just follow the steps as you recall them. For each exercise, prepare by arranging a yoga mat or blanket on the floor or on a firm surface. Put a pen and pad of paper (or your laptop computer) nearby. After you finish each exercise, record your thoughts. These recollections might be useful later, as you progress and improve in your visualization skills.

The Red Door

1. Lie down on your back in a comfortable place, in the Corpse pose (Chapter 8), with your arms slightly away from your body, palms facing up, legs relaxed, tailbone tucked under, shoulder blades tucked under, head and neck completely at rest. Close your eyes.

2. Inhale slowly and deeply, filling your lungs fully from the bottom, into the middle, and into the chest, to a count of 10. Hold your breath for three seconds at the top of the inhale. Then, exhale slowly and deeply over the count of ten. At the bottom of the exhale, hold your breath for one second.

3. Repeat this long slow breath seven times, continuing with short retentions after the inhalation and exhalation.

4. After the seventh breath, begin breathing normally, but imagine that all your breath flows in and out of your first chakra. Focus all your attention on the feel of that chakra.

5. Imagine you are standing in front of a white house with a red door. This might be a house you dream about sometimes, or a house you used to live in, or a house that you make up entirely, but it should feel comforting.

6. Walk up to the front door and look at the door. Notice what it looks like, how it is designed, what shape it is. Notice what kind of doorknob it has. Put your hand on the doorknob. Feel its weight and temperature and texture. Open the door and notice that it is a heavy, sturdy, secure door. Step into the house.

7. Inside, you see a room. Look around the room and notice what it looks like. Don't try to impose any qualities on the room, just look and see what you see in your mind's eye. As you look around, you notice a door on the far side of the room. Walk over to it and open it. You see a staircase with dim lights along the banister. Step onto the first stair and close the door behind you. There are seven stairs. Take a step down each until you reach the bottom.

8. At the bottom of the stairs, you find yourself in a dark room lit by a red glow. In the middle of the floor, you see a large circular pane of glass, about six feet in diameter, like a window in the floor. You walk over to it and look down. Behind the glass you see a deep, glittering, ruby-red wheel spinning, and you know this is your first chakra. Sit down on the floor and look at it for a while.

9. As you watch your chakra spinning, don't try to impose any thoughts or feelings on what you see. Just look and note the impressions that come to your mind. In particular, pay attention to the shade and brightness, size and shape, quality of the edges, speed and direction of the spin, and anything unusual you notice.

10. When you feel like you have looked long enough, imagine standing up, bowing to your first chakra, turning away, climbing the stairs, opening the door, walking through the main room, opening the front door, stepping out of the house, closing the door, turning to look at the red door, then walking away.

11. Slowly move your fingers and toes, bend your knees and hug them to your chest, roll over to your right side, and when you are ready, sit up and open your eyes.

Fire and Water

1. Sit comfortably on a folded blanket with your legs crossed. Breathe deeply in and out seven times, just as you did for the first exercise. When you have completed those seven breaths, begin breathing normally, but focus all your breath on your second chakra, as if you were breathing in and out from your abdomen.

2. Imagine walking through the woods at sunrise. The sun is just barely visible through the tree branches, which are losing their leaves. It is autumn and orange and yellow leaves flutter down from the trees and carpet the path so each step is cushioned and soft.

3. You come to a clearing next to a small stream. In the center of the clearing is a fire pit with a campfire burning brightly inside a circle of stones, as if it were waiting for you. You sit on a small log next to the fire, with the stream behind you.

4. Warm your hands at the fire, and throw sticks and leaves on it to keep it fueled. The fire makes you feel happy and content, and you stare at it, fascinated by the movement of the flames. You can hear the sound of the stream running over its rocky bed behind you. Watch the fire and listen to the stream.

5. As you continue to observe, the sound of the stream begins to combine with the sound of the fire, and the flames begin to change, melting down into each other and swirling into a bright orange eddy and then into what looks like a whirlpool of fire, right there on the forest floor. The spinning watery fire stays within the circle of rocks of the fire pit. You lean forward to watch it and you know it is your second chakra.

6. As with your first chakra, watch and notice the chakra's specific qualities.

7. When you think you have seen enough, stand, turn away, and walk back through the woods. When you are ready, gradually open your eyes.

Here Comes the Sun

Let your Power chakra help you visualize more intensely.

1. Sit comfortably on a folded blanket with your legs crossed. Breathe deeply in and out seven times, just as you did for the first exercise. Imagine your sitting bones grounding down into the earth, anchoring you safely.

2. When you have completed those seven breaths, begin breathing normally, but focus all your breath on your third chakra, as if you were breathing in and out from the base of your rib cage.

3. Imagine you are standing in a wide-open, rolling field of green grass on a sunny day. The sky is perfectly blue with no clouds and the sun has risen to about a 45-degree angle from the ground. Look all around you and notice everything you see.

4. Now look at the sun. It doesn't hurt your eyes and you can actually see its bright glowing golden shape. As you stare, you notice the sun is actually spinning like a spiral galaxy and you can see all the movements of fire and light on its surface as it spins. You know this is your third chakra, right out here in the open, beaming down on the world, unafraid.

5. As with your other chakras, watch and notice this chakra's shade and brightness, size and shape, speed and direction of spin, and anything unusual. Spend as much time as you need to observe, without judgment.

6. When you think you have seen enough, imagine lying down in the soft grass of the field and closing your eyes. Feel that sun on your skin and see its filtered light through your eyelids. What else do you see? What impressions, shapes, and forms swirl inside your inner vision?

7. When you are ready, gradually open your eyes.

Heart-Felt

Your Heart chakra can tell you a lot about yourself, so look closely!

1. Lie down on a yoga mat or a folded blanket in Corpse pose (Chapter 7). Breathe deeply in and out seven times, just as you did for the first exercise. When you have completed those seven breaths, begin breathing normally, but focus all your breath on your fourth chakra, as if you were breathing in and out from your heart.

2. Now, imagine you are walking through a city. The streets are busy with people walking and riding bicycles. Some people run, some stroll, but everybody is smiling or looking contented. You walk down a wide sidewalk, passing people who smile at you. The sidewalk isn't crowded but has a lively energy. Look around at all the people, the buildings, the lamp posts, the squares of the sidewalk, the

occasional trees and flowerbeds. Notice everything you can about this friendly city as you walk.

3. Now you see a glass building on your right, but the glass is fogged so you can't see what is inside. The building has an arched door painted bright green with a brass handle. Open the door and step inside.

4. You are inside a vast greenhouse. The vaulted ceiling is glass, and all the walls are glass. The air is humid and fragrant with the smell of greenery and flowers, and all around you are trees, vines, ferns, flowering bushes, and trays of seedlings. Look around.

5. You walk through the greenhouse to the other side, where you see there is another, smaller room, also made of glass. You step inside and see that the room is filled with orchids. In the middle of the room is a small fountain issuing steam. You walk between the tables with the trembling orchid flowers and step up to the fountain.

6. The fountain is set inside a wide silver bowl, about four feet in diameter. The jets quiet and as the spray falls back down into the water, the water in the base of the fountain begins to swirl like a whirlpool. You gaze into the fountain and you see the base is green with soft moss. The water swirls softly over the moss, and then it begins to take on the color of the moss until the swirling water becomes a swirling green light and you realize that this swirling fountain is your fourth chakra.

7. As with your other chakras, watch and notice this chakra's shade and brightness, size and shape, speed and direction of spin, and anything unusual. Spend as much time as you need to observe, without judgment.

8. When you think you have seen enough, step back from the fountain, turn, walk back out of the room full of orchids, back through the greenhouse, and back out the green door, onto the friendly street. When you are ready, gradually open your eyes.

To Tell the Truth

What truth can you tell from looking at your fifth chakra?

1. Sit comfortably on a folded blanket with your legs crossed. Breathe deeply in and out seven times, just as you did for the first exercise. Imagine your sitting bones

grounding down into the earth, anchoring you safely. When you have completed those seven breaths, begin breathing normally.

2. Imagine you are sitting in a tent. The wind blows the tent flaps open and shut and you can see the sun outside but inside the tent it is cool, dark, and calm. You sit on the ground and in front of you is a big blue crystal ball, about two feet in diameter, sitting on a solid granite pedestal. You gaze into the crystal ball and marvel at the swirling blue designs inside it.

3. You ask the crystal ball a question—anything you want to know. You stare into the crystal ball and you watch shapes and images begin to form. They speak to you and show you the answer to your question. The answer may not be direct or make sense right now, but just take it in.

4. After you've received an answer, look deep inside the crystal ball. The blue swirls begin to take form and organize, and they begin to rotate inside the crystal ball so that the entire inside of the crystal becomes a swirling wheel of blue energy. You realize that this is your fifth chakra.

5. As with your other chakras, watch and notice this chakra's qualities. When you think you have seen enough, stand up, turn away, and walk to the opening in the tent. Step out into the sun. When you are ready, gradually open your eyes.

Rest a little, or go on to the next exercise.

Third Eye on the Prize

Tap into your intuition by examining your sixth chakra.

1. Sit comfortably on a folded blanket with your legs crossed. Breathe deeply in and out seven times, just as you did for the first exercise. Imagine your sitting bones grounding down into the earth, anchoring you safely.

2. When you have completed those seven breaths, begin breathing normally, but focus all your breath on your sixth chakra, as if you were breathing in and out from your forehead.

3. Imagine you are standing in a dark room lit only by candles, in front of a huge mirror. The mirror has no frame. It is just a big piece of glass about the size of a large door, secured firmly against a wall. Step up to the mirror and look at yourself. Notice what you look like in this mirror.

4. Now, you notice a blue spot on your forehead. Step closer and look at your forehead in your reflection in the mirror. Look very closely. As you move closer, you see a dark, violet-blue spinning circle, right in the middle of your forehead. It begins to grow until it comes to its full size, and you know this is your sixth chakra. Examine it. See how it moves as you move, and expands when you stay still and breathe into it.

> **Energy Unplugged**
>
> The sixth chakra mirror exercise works for any of the chakras. You can visualize seeing them all in a mirror, one at a time, or even all at once. When you look at them all at once, you can compare and contrast their sizes, brightness, directions, and speeds of rotation.

5. As with your other chakras, watch and notice this chakra's shade and brightness, size and shape, speed and direction of spin, and anything unusual. Spend as much time as you need to observe, without judgment.

6. When you think you have seen enough, imagine placing your hand gently over your forehead. When you take your hand away, the chakra mark on your forehead is gone. Turn away from the mirror, and leave the room.

7. When you are ready, gradually open your eyes.

Rest a little, or go on to the next exercise.

Crowned

As usual, have a pen and paper or a computer handy for recording your impressions after you are finished.

1. Sit comfortably on a folded blanket with your legs crossed. Breathe deeply in and out seven times, just as you did for the first exercise. Imagine your sitting bones grounding down into the earth, anchoring you safely.

2. When you have completed those seven breaths, begin breathing normally, but focus all your breath on your seventh chakra, as if you were breathing in and out from the crown of your head.

3. Close your eyes and continue to breathe, but as you do, imagine that you are not breathing out of your own power. Imagine universal breath moving in and out of you, inhaling through the crown of your head as you exhale, exhaling into the crown of your head as you inhale.

4. Now breathe normally. Imagine yourself walking in a procession of finely dressed people down a deep purple carpet through a magnificent hall. As you walk, you realize the procession is centered around you. The people in front and behind are your guardians and people on either side of you cheer for you. You look down and see you are wearing a long robe covered in gold and silver embroidery and studded with beads and jewels. You continue to walk until you are led into a great room, up seven steps, and guided to sit on a beautiful throne.

5. You sit and the cushions of the throne are luxuriously comfortable and soft. You put your arms on the golden armrests, which are inlaid with pearls and diamonds. You run your hands over the jewels in the throne, then you look up and see that everyone is watching you and smiling with reverence and joy. What does the room look like? What do the people look like?

6. Now, a young boy walks toward you. He has pure white hair and pale skin and his eyes are a bright royal purple, unlike any eyes you've ever seen. He carries a purple cushion, and on it is a beautiful crown completely encrusted with diamonds. The diamonds sparkle with inner fire. He ascends the seven stairs and kneels before you, holding out the crown.

7. You lean over to look, and you see that inside the crown is a swirling white light. It grows and overtakes the crown, the cushion, and the boy so that all you see is this beautiful light. It rises up in front of you and turns so you can see it, spinning at your eye level about one foot in front of you. Look at it. Watch how it moves, what it looks like. You realize this is your seventh chakra.

8. As with your other chakras, watch and notice this chakra's shade and brightness, size and shape, speed and direction of spin, and anything unusual. Marvel at its pure beauty. Spend as much time as you need to observe, without judgment. Let the chakra live in front of you for as long as it likes.

9. When you think you have seen enough, reach your hands out and take the chakra. It solidifies again, becoming that diamond-encrusted crown. The boy is back, kneeling in front of you, holding the cushion, head bowed in respect. You place the crown on top of your head. Everyone in the room begins to applaud, but the applause grows fainter and fainter, and then the whole room disappears. All that is left is you, the crown, the breath, and light. Feel this and let it hold you, for as long as you like.

10. When you are ready, gradually open your eyes, stretch, and record all your impressions about your seventh chakra.

Understanding What You See

If you've done all seven exercises, you've made it to an important place. You've seen all your chakras. This is just the beginning, if you choose to continue working on this skill. You will eventually be able to go further, see more, and see your chakras more easily, with less visualization to set you up for seeing. Now, however, it's time to interpret what you have seen.

Remember that chakras can change from moment to moment, day to day. What you saw during your exercises are snapshots. It may be completely different the next time you look. As with measuring chakras, seeing chakras is most effective if you practice it on a regular basis. If one of your chakras is always smaller, or always spins counter-clockwise, or always has a dark spot in the lower left corner or a dent on the top, you have a chronic issue to deal with.

Look over your notes and notice which chakra seemed to be the brightest, the biggest, and the fastest-moving. These are likely to be your strongest, most open chakras. Notice which chakras seemed to be darker, smaller, or slower moving, or even not moving at all. These chakras are more likely to be your blocked chakras.

When chakras have holes or rips in them, you are having a problem in that chakra. You are missing something or have been hurt, or you might have a health issue related to that part of your body. The same holds true for dark spots, although these are more likely to be things in that part of your body or life that you don't want to see, so you are hiding them.

Chakras with wavering or blurry edges, especially if they are very large, may be over-loaded. Overloaded chakras also tend to move more slowly because they are having trouble processing all that energy.

When a chakra rotates counterclockwise, it may be regrouping, reenergizing, or purg-ing negative energy, which signifies healing. Or a counterclockwise rotating chakra may be blocked.

For quick reference, use this guide to interpret what you see, but also remember that a counterclockwise or dark or particularly slow or large chakra in *you* might not mean the same thing as it means in someone else. As you consider, even meditate, on what you see in your own chakras, keep asking yourself: *Does this feel true?* When it does feel true, when your interpretation resonates with your experience and you get that *a-ha* feeling, that's a thumbs-up sign from the universe that you're onto something.

Chakra Characteristics

Quality	Possible Meaning
Bright	Healthy
Dim	Blocked
Larger than other chakras	Overloaded
Smaller than other chakras	Blocked
Same size as other chakras	Healthy
Round	Healthy
Elliptical	In healing process or semi-blocked
Depressions or dents	Blocked
Bulges	Overloaded
Tears or rips	Sign of trauma or disease
Holes	Weak spots, insecurity in this area
Dark spots	Hiding some aspect from yourself
Wavy or blurry edges	Overloaded
Unevenness or anomalies on the top of the chakra	Problem with a spiritual or intellectual aspect of the area
Unevenness or anomalies on the bottom of the chakra	Problem with a physical / sensory or practical aspect of the area
Unevenness or anomalies on the right side of the chakra	Problem with yang / masculine energy related to the area
Unevenness or anomalies on the left side of the chakra	Problem with yin / feminine energy related to the area

continues

Chakra Characteristics (continued)

Quality	Possible Meaning
Faster spin than other chakras	Overloaded
Slower spin than other chakras	Blocked
Spin similar in speed to other chakras	Healthy
No spin/static	Blocked
Clockwise spin	Healthy
Counterclockwise spin	In healing process, purging negative energy, or blocked

Practicing yoga's Downward Facing Dog pose moves energy in the form of heat from the Heart chakra to your hands and feet. Visualizing this energy transfer while you hold the pose can help you to feel the release and flow of energy throughout your whole self.

Developing Your Chakra Vision

The more you work on seeing your chakras, the easier it gets. As you develop your skills, you use the exercises in this chapter to see all your chakras. For example, you could use the first exercise, going into the house with the red door, but make the door white. Go into different rooms in the downstairs of the house and see different lights in each room's floor, representing each chakra.

With regular practice, you can move beyond visualizations. During meditation, just focus in on each chakra and see it in your mind's eye. Eventually, you may even be able to look into a real full-length mirror at yourself and see your chakras. Keep practicing. Everybody has different ways of seeing, so when you find yours, there is no limit to what you will be able to see.

The Least You Need to Know

- You can actually learn to see your own chakras, rather than just imagining how they might look.

- Using chakra visualization techniques, you can diagnose the condition of your chakras, which can help you know what you need to get into better balance.

- When your chakra-seeing skills improve, you can check in with your chakras daily, as a way to monitor and improve your own well-being. You might even be able to see other people's chakras.

Chapter 20

More Than the Body You Can See

In This Chapter

♦ Three bodies, one you

♦ Your physical body

♦ Your astral body

♦ Your causal body

♦ Unity via the chakras

♦ Moving beyond yourself

Let's just say that you are so inspired by this book that you want to learn Sanskrit and fly off to India to study with a Tantric master. Fantastic. We're happy to have helped fuel your inspiration. However, we are guessing that, more likely, while you find chakra and yoga philosophy somewhat interesting, you are more interested in your chakras as a way to help you feel better and evolve in your personal life.

Either way, or even if you are somewhere between those two scenarios, we think you'll find this last short philosophical chapter interesting because it takes the theoretical concept of the chakras as well as the right-here, right-now reality of chakras beyond your body.

Actually, that's not entirely accurate. It takes the concept and reality of the chakras to the next *level* of your body—and the next level after that.

Your Three Bodies

You know all about your *physical body*, but did you know you also have an *astral body*, that permeates but extends slightly beyond your physical body? This is your energy body, and it is the realm of your *nadis* and your chakras. But your body-ness doesn't end there. You also have a *causal body*, and it permeates and extends beyond both your physical and astral bodies. It contains your soul. This is one of the basic ways that yoga philosophy understands the body.

def•i•ni•tion

The **physical body** is the body you can see and feel, comprised of your bones, muscles, organs, and physical features, as well as your physical feelings like pain and pleasure. The **astral body** permeates your physical body but extends up to about a foot beyond your physical body. This is your energy body and contains the *nadis*—energy channels—and chakras—energy vortexes where the *nadis* intersect. The **causal body** permeates the physical and astral bodies but extends to about a foot beyond your astral body. This is the realm of the soul and the essence of you that lives on when your physical body ceases to exist.

At least, that is a simplified explanation. We aren't going to bore you with the details of the entire cosmic infrastructure as yoga philosophy describes it. However, we do want to walk through the basics of the three bodies because understanding what they are, how they are different, how they interact with each other, and what they have to do with your chakras, can help you understand yourself better.

!!! Wake-Up Call

There are many different theories on the different subtle bodies, including how many there are and what they are called. Some theories, for example, name five bodies: the physical, etheric, astral, mental, and causal bodies. However, just as there are many chakras and we only discuss seven of them in this book, for our purposes, we have chosen to limit our discussion to the physical, astral, and causal bodies, with the full recognition that not everybody interprets things the same way we do, and not everyone who writes about such matters has learned about them from the same sources or traditions.

The Physical Body: Blood, Guts, and Glory

We don't have to introduce you to your physical body. You already know it well. This body is made up of your bones, muscles, organs, and blood. The physical body has legs and arms, a torso, a face, hair, fingernails, and toenails and teeth. This is the body that gets headaches and pulled muscles, that loves to eat and sleep and have sex. This body breathes air, drinks water, and needs to sleep. It is the body you see when you look in the mirror.

The chakras don't live in the physical body, which is why you can't see them. You can see the parts of the physical body, inside and out, either with the naked eye, with a microscope, or with medical equipment like x-ray machines and MRIs. Yet chakras exist within (and outside of) the physical body, and structures within the physical body, such as clusters of nerves, particular glands, and certain organs, relate to and respond to the energy of the chakras.

The Astral Body: *Prana* Central

Your physical body breathes in air, but with every breath, the astral body also breathes in *prana*. The astral body permeates the physical body and exists inside of it, but it is also bigger than the physical body and extends anywhere from a few inches up to about a foot beyond the physical body. You move your arm, and your astral body's "arm" moves, too, as the energy imprint and aura of the physical body's arm.

The astral body is your energy body. It is the realm of thought and also the place where *prana* moves through you, in and out of you. This is the body that contains the meridians doctors use for acupuncture and Shiatsu massage. They put needles in and press points on your physical body, but they are doing it in order to manipulate the energy flow within your astral body.

Spinning Your Wheels

Some people practice astral projection, a conscious and purposeful out-of-body experience in which the astral body leaves the physical body for a while. This is a difficult practice that not everyone is able to master, although some people crave it and strive for it. Others believe astral projection doesn't exist and is really just dreaming. There is a tradition of astral projection in certain cultures, such as among certain Native American tribes, but like all other aspects of the astral body, the phenomenon can't be measured or proven using society's current tools and techniques, which are limited to the phenomena of the physical body.

The astral body contains not just the primary meridians but thousands and thousands of energy channels like a network of rivers and streams on a planet. At every intersection between two or more energy channels, there exists a chakra. Although this book focuses on the seven primary chakras along the midline of the body, there are thousands of other chakras of various sizes and strengths, all over the body.

Because your chakras exist in the astral rather than the physical body, you can't see them through normal visual means (see Chapter 19). However, they are hard at work bringing *prana* into your body and processing it. This is *prana* transforming your physical qualities into energy, which your chakras process and then respond to by getting bigger or smaller, brighter or dimmer, or changing shape or speed. Once the chakras process what is going on in your physical body, those events become a part of your energy body and a part of your thoughts, feelings, and the energetic expression of yourself.

The astral body is also the source of your *aura*, which is the part of your astral body that extends beyond your physical body. In the same way that you can learn to see the chakras, you can also learn to see your aura, and the auras of others.

def•i•ni•tion

The **aura** is the energy field in and around every person or object, and the outer boundary of the astral or energetic body, which is larger than the physical body. Some people believe auras can be photographed using a technique called Kirlian photography, although not everybody agrees that a Kirlian image really does show the aura.

Seeing auras is interesting, and a great way to get a sense of the astral body. It is also (arguably) easier than seeing chakras. The auras encircle all people and objects like a whole-body halo. We could write a whole separate book about auras and using them to diagnose problems and improve your life, but for now, we'll just say that people have auras of different sizes, shapes, and colors, and like chakras, auras can change depending on what you are doing, feeling, thinking, and experiencing. If you stand in front of a mirror and relax your eyes, you may be able to see your aura. If you practice, you may eventually begin noticing other people's auras.

The Causal Body: Universal You

The causal body permeates and interpenetrates the physical and astral bodies but extends beyond these bodies to form a sort of egg shape around you that extends approximately two or three feet beyond your physical body. The causal body carries the seed energy of *you*, which some people think of as the soul.

Even when your physical body is gone and your astral body dissipates into the ether, your causal body remains.

According to the *Law of Karma*, the causal body carries on into the next *reincarnation*. It will take the form of a new physical and astral body, but the causal body will be the same. Karma is commonly discussed in terms of past lives because the actions of an individual can become imprinted on the causal body and the individual can carry that imprint from one life to the next, so that what happens in one life can be the reaction to what happened in a previous life.

def•i•ni•tion

The **Law of Karma** is an ancient Eastern concept that says, in essence, that there is no good or bad, only action and reaction, or cause and effect. Everything you do, and everything that happens, is imprinted on the universe and will eventually be balanced by other actions or happenings. **Reincarnation** is the belief that the soul is reborn many times into different physical bodies.

Although the chakras exist within the astral body, they are also a link between the physical and causal bodies because the result of *prana* processed through the chakras is part of the imprint upon the causal body. In other words, all three bodies are linked, and what links them most potently are the energy vortexes that are the chakras.

How Your Chakras Bring Your Bodies Together

When we envision the three bodies—physical, overlain by astral, overlain by causal— we like to think of the chakras as a row of buttons down the middle, holding them all together. The physical body is like the bottom layer of clothes and the causal body is like the top layer. The astral body floats between them, with the chakras buttoning them all together into one whole being: you.

Understanding that you are more than your physical body—that your energy has a body and your soul has a body, too—can help you to understand how much bigger and more important you are than you might have thought—and what potential you have for evolution. Your chakras anchor you to that something bigger. They are the means for accomplishing a better, more complex, more amazing, and eventually enlightened you.

Sure, it's all a bit esoteric, but think of it like this: you are more than your physical body. You are more than your thoughts. You are more than your soul. But you are all those things, and the common thread between them all is the thread running from the base of your spine to the crown of your head.

Connecting to your partner's chakra energy means joining your astral and causal bodies as well as your physical ones.

Your chakras help to take a piece of universal consciousness and mold it into an individual body-mind-spirit. You are here, now, for a reason, and your chakras are here to help you figure out what that reason is.

Life is funny. It is so full of challenges, pain, and separation, but also so full of connection, beauty, and joy. Life isn't meant to be easy, but it is a gift that we get to be here, inhabiting these bodies on this beautiful earth for a little while, and so fortuitous that we have our very own chakras as tools to make the most of our lives. And when do we finally make the most of it? In this lifetime, or over the course of a thousand lifetimes? The point is that we have the opportunity to make the most of it, and having our seven chakras (and all the others) is part of that opportunity. So what are you waiting for?

Stepping Into Love

The end goal of our journey on this earth and through this life, according to yoga, is to finally fully understand that we are part of universal consciousness—an integral part. When we see that, when we have finally learned all the lessons we come here to learn, we take the final step: we move out of ourselves and into love. Finally, in the end, we get to turn in those bodies—all three of them—and drop back down like a wave rolling up a beach and falling back into the ocean.

You don't have to believe in reincarnation to understand the chakras, but if you do believe in reincarnation, you can see that you could live a thousand lives in a thousand physical bodies with a thousand different sets of chakras, all plugging away to make it work—to help you *see*. When you've learned everything you need to learn, at long last, you get to go home to the universal consciousness where you started. Maybe this is how the universe itself evolves, tiny bit by tiny bit, part by part, or heart by heart.

Or maybe you don't believe in reincarnation. It doesn't matter because where the chakras are concerned, it comes to the same thing. You are here, inside layers of bodies and layers of meaning, feeling, and understanding. You are right here, right now, in order to learn how to be something bigger than yourself—to remember who you really are. The chakras spin and churn and process your energy to help you see the truth. When you finally do, you get to step back out of those bodies—those temporary tools—back into the great current of love. You were born there, and in the end, it's where you belong.

You hold within you the sun and the moon and all of the universe. As you join your palms in yoga's Prayer pose, inhale and feel prana flow to your Heart chakra. As you exhale, feel that energy flow toward heaven and Earth. Namaste. We honor the divine light within you.

The chakras are such powerful tools for this ultimate process of transformation that we sincerely hope you will continue to work on them, feel them, measure them, look at them, contemplate them, and heal them. We believe that only through the evolution of one person here, one person there, each person at a time, will the human race ever really move to the next level of consciousness and awareness. We see a future that sparkles with promise and glows with hope, and it is a future that you can help grow.

And we'll help. We can all help grow the future of the human race together because when we change ourselves, we change the world. Happiness, peace, and love are powerful and infectious. When you find them within yourself, they radiate from your life, from your chakras, from your very pores, and everyone around you feels the difference. Let your chakras help you become that difference, and we promise to keep working on ourselves, too.

The light within us recognizes and honors the light within you. May we all go forth, secure in our first chakras, passionate in our second chakras, powerful in our third chakras, loving in our fourth chakras, truthful in our fifth chakras, intuitive in our sixth chakras, and filled with the bliss that flows into our seventh chakras from the love that catalyzed us.

And may we shine.

The Least You Need to Know

- Every person has a physical body that you can see, an astral body that is the realm of energy and the chakras, and a causal body that houses the soul and lives on after the physical body dies.

- The chakras tie all three bodies together by taking information from the physical body, transforming it via the chakras into thoughts and feelings, and imprinting that individuality upon the causal body.

- When we finally learn all the lessons we are meant to learn and recognize that we are part of the divine force of universal love, we can leave all three of our bodies and return to the universal energy that created us, like a wave falling back into the sea.

Glossary

Are you wondering what the heck we're talking about? Find those obscure or technical words here.

ahimsa   One of the *yamas*, which make up the first of the Eight Limbs of Yoga as described by Patanjali in the *Yoga Sutras*. To practice *ahimsa* is to abstain from violence.

Air chakra   See *Anahata*.

Ajna   Commanding, perceiving, or understanding in Sanskrit, pronounced *aj*-nyah, this is the sixth chakra, also called the Third Eye chakra, Intuition chakra, or Psychic chakra. Located just above the area between the eyebrows, this chakra controls intuition, reflection, inner knowledge, perception, and clairvoyance, or psychic "seeing."

Alzheimer's disease   The most common cause of dementia in older people, Alzheimer's disease is a progressive brain disease that gradually destroys memory and cognitive abilities. It is most common in people over 60 years old.

Anahata   Intact or unstruck in Sanskrit, pronounced ah-*nah*-ha-tah, this is the fourth chakra, also called the Heart chakra, Love chakra, or Air chakra. It is located in front of the heart. This chakra rules love, compassion, empathy, and your social sense of self.

aparigraha   One of the *yamas*, which make up the first of the Eight Limbs of Yoga as described by Patanjali in the *Yoga Sutras*. To practice *aparigraha* is to abstain from being jealous and to abstain from coveting what others have.

asana   One of the Eight Limbs of Yoga, as described by Patanjali in the *Yoga Sutras*. *Asana* is pronounced *ah*-sah-nah, and is discipline of the body through yoga poses. The poses themselves are called *asanas*.

asteya   One of the *yamas*, which make up the first of the Eight Limbs of Yoga as described by Patanjali in the *Yoga Sutras*. To practice *asteya* is to abstain from stealing.

atheism   The belief that there is no God or higher power beyond nature.

atheist   Someone who believes there is no God or higher power.

AUM   The sound representing the sixth chakra. This is also the sound of the seventh chakra when spoken by God or perceived through universal vibration rather than spoken by a person. See also *Om*.

autism   A mental disorder with onset prior to 3 years of age, that is marked by impaired development in social interaction and communication, and a restricted repertoire of activity and interests.

Balasana   The Sankrit term for Child's pose, a restorative yoga pose involving kneeling and resting the torso and head on the ground.

bandha   The Sanskrit word for lock, these are muscular contractions of the body practiced to hold energy or *prana* inside the body temporarily. There are three primary *bandhas: mula bandha, uddiyana bandha,* and *jalandhara bandha*.

Bhujangasana   The Sanskrit term for Cobra pose, a yoga pose involving lying on the stomach while raising the head and chest off the floor. This pose is good for many chakras, including the first and the fourth.

Bikram yoga   See *Hot yoga*.

bipolar disorder   A mental disorder characterized by mood swings, ranging from depression to mania (abnormally elevated, expansive or irritable mood).

Boat pose   See *Navasana*.

brahmacharya   One of the *yamas*, which make up the first of the Eight Limbs of Yoga as described by Patanjali in the *Yoga Sutras*. To practice *brahmacharya* is to abstain from sexual misconduct.

Bridge pose   See *Setu Bandha*.

Buddhism   A religion that began in India over 2,000 years ago with a man named Siddhartha Gautama, who became enlightened and is now known as the Buddha. Today, millions of people all over the world practice any of several branches of Buddhism, but Buddhism is more widespread in Asia.

bulimia   An eating disorder characterized by repeated episodes of binge-eating followed by inappropriate compensatory behaviors such as self-induced vomiting, misuse of laxatives, fasting, or excessive exercise.

caduceus   A Greek symbol used today to represent the practice of medicine, it depicts a staff with two snakes entwining around it from bottom to top. This symbol is often used to describe the way in which the masculine and feminine energy channels or *nadis* coil around a central energy channel in the body, called *sushumna nadi*, which runs along the spinal column.

cakra   The original spelling of *chakra*.

cakravartins   The Sanskrit name for the Aryans that invaded India during the Indo-European invasion.

Camel pose   See *Ustrasana*.

cardiac nerve plexus   A cluster of nerves associated with the fourth or Heart chakra.

chakras   Chakra is the Sanskrit term for wheel. Pronounced cha-kra, with a hard "ch" like in "chair," chakras are spinning energy centers in the body that lie along the body's many energy pathways. While chakras correspond to certain glands, nerve centers, and organs in the body, they are part of the subtle energy body, not the physical body, so they cannot be detected by standard medical equipment like X-rays or MRIs. Chakras also correspond to various aspects of the body's physical, psychological, emotional, and spiritual state.

chi   The Chinese term for the same life force energy that is *prana*, and the term acupuncturists, Shiatsu massage therapists, and other energy healers often use. *Prana* and *chi* are essentially the same thing, going by different names because they came from different languages.

Child's pose   See *Balasana*.

Cobra pose   See *Bhujangasana*.

coccygeal nerve plexus   The cluster of nerves associated with the first chakra.

codependency A psychological term used to describe a relationship pattern in which someone becomes so preoccupied with giving to and caring for someone else that they neglect themselves. The codependent person believes that something or someone outside of themselves will make them fulfilled and happy. To these people, life is only okay if those around them are happy and well, thanks to their actions and care.

Communication chakra See *Vishuddha*.

Corpse pose See *Savasana*.

Crown chakra See *Sahasrara*.

Dandasana Staff pose, a basic sitting yoga pose.

dementia The impairment of daily living skills like memory, attention, orientation, judgment, language, and motor skills, to the point that it interferes with normal functioning.

dharana One of the Eight Limbs of Yoga, as described by Patanjali in the *Yoga Sutras*. *Dharana* is concentration.

dharma wheel See *dharmachakra*.

dharmachakra The Sanskrit word for dharma wheel, this is a symbol of a wheel with eight spokes representing each limb of the Noble Eightfold Path of Buddhism.

dhyana One of the Eight Limbs of Yoga, as described by Patanjali in the *Yoga Sutras*. *Dhyana* is meditation.

Eagle pose See *Garudasana*.

Earth chakra See *Muladhara*.

Eight Limbs of Yoga Eight steps or parts of yoga, as described by *Patanjali* in the *Yoga Sutras*. The eight limbs include *yamas* (abstaining from violence, lying, stealing, sexual misconduct, and coveting), *niyamas* (practicing cleanliness, satisfaction, self-discipline, study, and worship of God or surrender to a higher power), *asana* (discipline of the body through yoga poses), *pranayama* (breath control), *pratyahara* (sensory withdrawal), *dharana* (concentration), *dhyana* (meditation), and *samadhi* (experiencing the unity of all things).

Eightfold Path The fourth of the Four Noble Truths of Buddhism. It consists of guidelines for living that help increase knowledge and maximize the chances for enlightenment. The eight paths are right understanding, right thought, right speech, right action, right livelihood, right effort, right mindfulness, and right concentration.

The Noble Eightfold Path is often represented by a wheel or chakra called the *dharma wheel* or *dharmachakra* in Sanskrit. This is a symbol of a wheel with eight spokes representing each limb of the Noble Eightfold Path.

fifth chakra   See *Vishuddha*.

first chakra   See *Muladhara*.

Fish pose   See *Matsyasana*.

Four Noble Truths   A concept central to Buddhist thought that covers the main problems humans encounter, and what to do about them. The Four Noble Truths are: 1) Life entails suffering; 2) Suffering is caused by desire; 3) We can eliminate suffering by eliminating desire; and 4) Adhering to the Eightfold Path is the key to eliminating desire, and thereby eliminating suffering.

HANG   The sound representing the fifth chakra.

Hatha yoga   A type of yoga popular in the world today that emphasizes physical poses, or *asanas*, to gain mastery over the body.

headstand   See *Sirsanana*.

Heart chakra   See *Anahata*.

Hinduism   A religion that began in India thousands of years ago and is one of the oldest known religions. Today it is the third largest religion in the world, after Christianity and Islam. Yoga was originally a part of the Hindu tradition, although today, yoga—primarily Hatha yoga—is practiced by millions of people who are not Hindu.

Hot yoga   Hot yoga is practiced in a room typically heated to around 100 degrees, with high humidity, similar to the climate in India, where yoga originated. This type of yoga induces sweating to purge toxins from the body. The heat also increases flexibility. *Bikram* is the most well-known style of hot yoga.

hypnosis   A state of altered consciousness during which there is increased focus and a greater openness to suggestion.

ida nadi   The energy channel that carries feminine energy from the base of the spine, coiling around the spine in opposition to *pingala nadi*, and ending at the crown.

Intuition chakra   See *Ajna*.

ishvarapranidhana   One of the *niyamas*, which make up the second of the Eight Limbs of Yoga, as described by Patanjali in the *Yoga Sutras*. To practice *ishvarapranidhana* is to worship God or surrender to a higher power.

jhalandara bandha   The Sanskrit term for the throat lock, an action to hold energy in the body by closing the throat for a few seconds after inhaling. This is particularly energizing for the fifth chakra. This *bandha* is often used in conjunction with *uddiyana bandha*, to hold energy inside the body.

Kundalini   A Sanskrit term meaning "coiled one," *Kundalini* is an ancient yoga concept that feminine energy lies coiled like a serpent at the base of the spine inside the first chakra. As *Kundalini* energy is awakened, she desires to merge with masculine energy (sometimes represented as the Hindu god Shiva) so she rises up through each chakra, activating that chakra. The result is gradual awakening.

LANG   The sound representing the first chakra.

Love chakra   See *Anahata*.

mahat   A Sanskrit term for the element associated with the sixth chakra. *Mahat* means "supreme element" and is a sort of super element that is a combination of all the other elements.

mandala   A picture of a wheel-like design similar to a chakra, for focusing the mind during meditation.

Manipura   Dwelling place for the jewel or city of the jewel in Sanskrit, pronounced mah-nee-*poo*-rah, this is the third chakra, also called the Power chakra, Sun chakra, or Solar Plexus chakra, located in that space just below the midline of the rib cage, at the solar plexus. This chakra governs your personal power, sense of self, willpower, and digestion.

mantra   The Sanskrit word for a sacred syllable or phrase that is spoken repeatedly during meditation, to aid in concentration and focus.

mantra meditation   A form of meditation in which a *mantra*—a sound or phrase—is spoken repeatedly, to aid in concentration and focus. Mantra meditation is particularly good for energizing the fifth or Throat chakra.

martyr complex   A psychological term referring to a relationship pattern where a person, the martyr, suffers on purpose, often in the name of helping or serving someone else, suffering for love, or suffering for a cause, at the expense of personal needs or desires. The martyr often becomes resentful because the love they shower on others isn't returned to them in the way they want.

Matsyasana   The Sanskrit word for the Fish pose in yoga, a pose involving lying on the back with the crown of the head tipped back to touch the floor. This pose is good for opening and energizing both the fifth or Throat chakra and the seventh or Crown chakra.

medical intuitive A person with the ability to use their own intuition to determine specific physical, emotional, or psychological illnesses or imbalances in another person. Sometimes medical intuitives "see" a specific problem, such as a cancerous tumor in a particular place. Sometimes they simply get a sense of what the problem is, or even feel the same pain in their own bodies.

meditation A mental technique for quieting and focusing the mind, for stress relief, relaxation, solving problems, or to move toward enlightenment.

mindfulness meditation A type of meditation that helps you to focus on the present moment without getting caught up in mental trips to the past or future. Typically, the technique for beginning mindfulness meditation is to focus on the breath, to help the mind stay in the present moment.

Mountain pose See *Tadasana*.

mudras A Sanskrit word referring (most commonly) to specific hand and finger positions that affect the internal energy of the body in specific ways. They are used in several ancient Eastern traditions, including yoga and Buddhism.

mula bandha The Sanskrit term for the root lock, an action to hold energy in the body by contracting the muscles at the floor of the pelvis. This *bandha* energizes and opens the first or Root chakra.

Muladhara Root or base support in Sanskrit, pronounced moo-*lah*-de-har-uh, this is the first chakra, also called the Earth or Root chakra, located at the base of the spine, just in front of the tailbone. This chakra keeps you grounded in your physical body and governs your sense of security, survival, safety, and physical identity.

nadi A channel in the body through which *prana* or life force energy flows. Acupuncturists and other healers use the *nadis* to help free life force energy in the body for enhanced healing.

narcissism A psychological term referring to a personality characteristic in which there is excessive self-importance and a need for constant admiration, to such an extent that the narcissistic person is not able to love or feel empathy for others.

Navasana The Sanskrit word for Boat pose, a seated balancing yoga pose.

niyamas One of the limbs of the Eight Limbs of Yoga, as described by Patanjali in the *Yoga Sutras*. The *niyamas* consist of five observances: *shaucha* (cleanliness), *santosha* (satisfaction), *tapas* (self-discipline), *svadhyaya* (study), and *ishvarapranidhana* (worship of God or surrender to a higher power).

Noble Eightfold Path See *Eightfold Path*.

Om   Sometimes spelled *AUM*, *Om* is a sacred symbol in Hinduism, representing the impersonal, omnipotent, absolute source of all creation. According to Hindu thought, the sound of *Om* encompasses the past, present, and future and was the original vibration that created the universe. It is often used as a mantra in meditation or prayer and speaking; this intonation is thought to penetrate the soul. See also *AUM*.

Passion chakra   See *Svadhisthana*.

Patanjali   A man who lived in India in about the second century B.C.E., who compiled the Yoga Sutras, a collection of aphorisms distilling the essence of what yoga is.

pharyngeal nerve plexus   The cluster of nerves associated with the fifth chakra.

Pilates   A form of exercise that develops core strength, or the muscular strength of the abdominal and back muscles. Pilates exercises traditionally use a specific machine designed for the purpose, but can also be adapted for mat exercises, without any equipment. Pilates classes are widely available at health clubs, yoga studios, and elsewhere.

pingala nadi   The energy channel that carries masculine energy from the base of the spine, coiling around the spine in opposition to *ida nadi*, and ending at the crown.

PMS   An acronym for premenstrual syndrome, a condition triggered by hormonal changes that typically occurs one to two weeks before menstruation, characterized by emotional and physical symptoms like mood swings, irritability, bloating, and food cravings.

Power chakra   See *Manipura*.

prana   The Sanskrit term for life force energy, *prana* flows into and out of the body with the breath and through the chakras via channels in the body called *nadis*. The Chinese term for life force energy is *chi*. *Prana* and *chi* are essentially the same thing, going by different names because they came from different languages.

prana mudra   A mudra that joins the index and little finger tips with the thumb, to re-route *prana* back into the body for greater healing.

pranayama   One of the Eight Limbs of Yoga, as described by Patanjali in the *Yoga Sutras*. *Pranayama* is the practice of breath control.

pratyahara   The yogic principle of withdrawing the senses from external objects to focus on the inner vision. This is one of the Eight Limbs of Yoga, as described by Patanjali in the *Yoga Sutras*. Regular sensory withdrawal results in greater control over the senses, so they are not mistaken for more than they are.

projection   The psychological term for seeing qualities or problems in others that we are actually experiencing ourselves.

Psychic chakra   See *Ajna*.

psychosis   A mental disorder characterized by failure to recognize what is real and what is not real, to the extent that the psychotic person has difficulty meeting the demands of everyday life. Symptoms can include hallucinations, delusions, and paranoia.

RANG   The sound representing the third chakra.

Root chakra   See *Muladhara*.

Sacral Chakra   See *Svadhisthana*.

sacral nerve plexus   The cluster of nerves associated with the second chakra.

Sahasrara   Thousand-petaled or thousand-spoked in Sanskrit, pronounced sah-hah-*srah*-rah, this is the seventh chakra, also called the Crown chakra, Spiritual chakra, or Thousand-Petaled Lotus chakra. It is located at the crown of the head. This is our gateway to wisdom, enlightenment, and the knowledge that we are one with all things. It is our link to divinity and to our own intellect.

samadhi   One of the Eight Limbs of Yoga, as described by Patanjali in the *Yoga Sutras*. *Samadhi* is the experience of the unity of all things.

Sanskrit   One of the ancient languages of India. The *Vedas*—the first written texts in India—were written in Sanskrit. Sanskrit is most commonly known today due to its association with the yoga tradition.

santosha   One of the *niyamas*, which make up the second of the Eight Limbs of Yoga, as described by Patanjali in the *Yoga Sutras*. To practice *santosha* is to be content.

satya   One of the *yamas*, which make up the first of the Eight Limbs of Yoga as described by Patanjali in the *Yoga Sutras*. To practice *satya* is to abstain from lying.

Savant Syndrome   An unofficial term for a condition in which someone has highly advanced skills in one area such as art, math, music, or remembering dates, usually in conjunction with a mental disability such as autism.

Savasana   Corpse pose, a restorative yoga pose involving lying on the floor, face up, and relaxing completely.

second chakra   See *Svadhisthana*.

Setu Bandha   The Sanskrit term for Bridge pose, a yoga pose involving lying on the back while raising the hips and chest. This pose is good for energizing the fourth chakra.

seventh chakra   See *Sahasrara*.

sexual arousal disorder   A disorder characterized by the inability to become aroused, sustain arousal, or experience orgasm during sexual activity. This can happen to men or women, and may have physical or psychological causes. In either case, this disorder is reflected in a blocked second chakra.

Sexual chakra   See *Svadhisthana*.

Shakti   A Hindu goddess that represents the female principle. When paired with Shiva, the male element, they represent the Divine. The word is also sometimes used to refer to divine creative power. *Kundalini* energy is sometimes associated with Shakti. As *Kundalini* energy moves through the chakras, she is moving upward to join with Shiva in ultimate union, a symbolic description of enlightenment.

shaucha   One of the *niyamas*, which make up the second of the Eight Limbs of Yoga, as described by Patanjali in the *Yoga Sutras*. To practice *shauca* is to purify the body.

Shiva   A Hindu god that represents the ultimate male principle. When paired with Shakti, the female element, they represent the Divine.

Sirsana   The Sanskrit name for Headstand pose.

sixth chakra   See *Ajna*.

solar plexus   The cluster of nerves associated with the third chakra.

Solar Plexus chakra   See *Manipura*.

Spiritual chakra   See *Sahasrara*.

Staff pose   See *Dandasana*.

Sun chakra   See *Manipura*.

Surya Namaskar   The Sanskrit name for sun salutation, a sequence of 12 yoga poses. The sequence is meant to be practiced in the morning, as a ritual for warming up the body and saluting the rising sun.

sushumna nadi   The central *nadi* or energy channel in the body, running along the spinal column from the first to the seventh chakra. The seven primary chakras are lined up along the *sushumna nadi* and *ida nadi* and *pingala nadi* coil around this central channel like the double helix of DNA or that symbol of medicine, the caduceus (two snakes coiled around a staff).

Svadhisthana   Dwelling place of the self of sweetness in Sanskrit, pronounced swa-dee-*shtah*-nuh, this is the second chakra, also called the Passion, Sexual, or Sacral chakra, located just below the naval, in front of the sacrum. This chakra governs your emotions, passions, creativity, fertility, and sexuality.

svadhyaya One of the *niyamas*, which make up the second of the Eight Limbs of Yoga, as described by Patanjali in the *Yoga Sutras*. To practice *svadhyaya* is to study.

Tadasana Mountain pose, a basic standing yoga pose.

Tantra A branch of the yoga tradition often associated with sexual practices, but this is a misunderstanding of this esoteric form of yoga. According to Tantra, our sensory experience and the physical universe itself is a manifestation of divine energy, and so should be celebrated, rather than transcended. An essential part of Tantra is the concept of *Kundalini*.

tapas One of the *niyamas*, which make up the second of the Eight Limbs of Yoga, as described by Patanjali in the *Yoga Sutras*. To practice *tapas* is to be self-discliplined.

Third Eye chakra See *Ajna*.

Thousand-Petaled Lotus chakra See *Sahasrara*.

Throat chakra See *Vishuddha*.

Tree pose See *Vrksasana*.

Truth chakra See *Vishuddha*.

uddiyana bandha The Sanskrit term for the abdominal lock, an action to hold energy in the body by pulling the abdominal muscles in and upward and holding them, to concentrate energy in the third or Solar Plexus chakra. This *bandha* is often used in conjunction with *jhalandara bandha*, to hold energy inside the body.

Upanishads Hindu scriptures sacred to the Vedanta branch of Hinduism.

Ustrasana The Sanskrit word for Camel pose, a back-bending pose involving kneeling and reaching back to grasp the feet. This pose is good for opening and energizing the fifth or Throat chakra.

VANG The sound representing the second chakra.

Vedas The very first written texts in India that consist of a huge body of literature, probably dating back to 2000 B.C.E. Orthodox Hindus consider the *Vedas* to be sacred texts inspired by God.

Vinyasa A Sanskrit word commonly used to describe a style of Hatha yoga that links sequences of poses together in a flowing motion, rather than holding poses for long periods.

Virabhadrasana I The Sanskrit word for Warrior I pose, an energizing, standing yoga pose.

Virabhadrasana II   The Sanskrit word for Warrior II pose, an energizing, standing yoga pose.

Virabhadrasana III   The Sanskrit word for Warrior III pose, a yoga standing balance pose.

Vishuddha   Purity in Sanskrit, pronounced vee-*shoo*-duh, this is the fifth chakra, also called the Truth chakra, Throat chakra, or Communication chakra. It is located in the hollow of the throat between the inner edges of the collarbone. This chakra controls communication, creativity, the use of language and symbolic thought, and the ability to speak and hear the truth.

visualization   The act of forming mental images or pictures in one's mind for various purposes like relaxation, skill enhancement, or healing.

Vrksasana   Tree pose, a balancing yoga pose.

Warrior I   See *Virabhadrasana I.*

Warrior II   See *Virabhadrasana II.*

Warrior III   See *Virabhadrasana III.*

yamas   One of the Eight Limbs of Yoga, as described by Patanjali in the *Yoga Sutras.* The *yamas* consist of healthy practices to guide moral life: *ahimsa* (non-violence), *satya* (truthfulness), *asteya* (non-stealing), *brahmacharya* (abstaining from sexual misconduct), and *aparigraha* (not being jealous or coveting what others have).

YANG   The sound representing the fourth chakra.

yoga   A Sanskrit word meaning "to yoke," yoga is an ancient practice originating in India with the purpose of yoking or unifying the body, mind, and spirit. Yoga involves many practices including physical postures, called *asanas;* meditation; breathing exercises called *pranayama;* and ethical guidelines for living. Today, yoga is most often used to describe Hatha yoga, a form of yoga that primarily emphasizes the physical poses or *asanas.*

Yoga Sutras   An important yoga text written by Patanjali in the second century, consisting of aphorisms that distill the essence of yoga, including the Eight Limbs of Yoga.

zazen   A Zen Buddhist meditation technique, zazen means "just sitting."

Resources

If you enjoyed this book and you would like to read more about chakras, yoga, energy healing, and the other subjects covered in this book, we recommend the following resources, all of which one or both of us have read and used over the years.

Ashley-Farrand, Thomas. *Chakra Mantras: Liberate your spiritual genius through chanting*. San Francisco, CA, Weiser Books, 2006.

Bachman, Nicolai. *The Language of Yoga: Complete A to Y guide to asana names, Sanskrit terms, and chants*. Boulder, CO: Sounds True, 2004.

Brennan, Barbara Ann. *Hands of Light: A guide to healing through the human energy field*. New York, NY: Bantam Books, 1987.

Dale, Cyndi. *Advanced Chakra Healing: Energy mapping on the four pathways*. Berkeley, CA: The Crossing Press, 2005.

Davies, Brenda. *The 7 Healing Chakras: Unlocking your body's energy centers*. Berkeley, CA: Ulysses Press, 2007

Eden, Donna, with David Feinstein. *Energy Medicine*. New York, NY: Jeremy P. Tarcher/Putnam, 1998.

Gerber, Richard, M.D. *A Practical Guide to Vibrational Medicine: Energy healing and spiritual transformation.* New York, NY: Quill, 2001.

Govinda, Kalashatra. *A Handbook of Chakra Healing: Spiritual practice for health, harmony, and inner peace.* Old Saybrook, CT: Konecky & Konecky, 2002.

Iyengar, B.K.S. *Light on Pranayama: The yogic art of breathing.* New York, NY: The Crossroad Publishing Company, 2008.

———. *Light on Yoga.* New York, NY: Schocken Books, 1966.

Johari, Harish. *Chakras: Energy centers of transformation.* Rochester, VT: Destiny Books, 2000.

Judith, Anodea. *Chakra Balancing: A guide to healing and awakening your energy body.* Boulder, CO: Sounds True, 2003.

———. *Eastern Body, Western Mind: Psychology and the chakra system as a path to the self, revised.* Berkeley, CA: Celestial Arts, 2004.

———. *Wheels of Life: A User's Guide to the Chakra System.* Woodbury, MN: Llewellyn Publications, 1999.

McCall, Timothy, M.D. *Yoga as Medicine: The yogic prescription for health and healing.* New York, NY: Bantam Books, 2007.

McLaren, Karla. *Your Aura & Your Chakras: An owner's manual.* York Beach, ME: Weiser Books, 1998.

Mumford, Dr. Jonn. *A Chakra & Kundalini Workbook, 4th edition expanded.* Woodbury, MN: Llewellyn Publications, 2008.

Myss, Caroline, Ph.D. *Anatomy of the Spirit: The seven stages of power and healing.* New York, NY: Three Rivers Press, 1996.

Northrup, Christiane, M.D. *Women's Bodies, Women's Wisdom: Creating physical and emotional health and healing.* New York, NY: Bantam Books, 1998.

Selby, John. *Kundalini Awakening: A Gentle Guide to Chakra Activation and Spiritual Growth*. New York, NY: Bantam Books, 1992.

Wauters, Ambika. *Chakras and Their Archetypes: Uniting energy awareness and spiritual growth*. Berkeley, CA: The Crossing Press, 1997.

Index

D

E

T